THE EYE OF REVELATION

1939 & 1946 EDITIONS COMBINED

The True Five Tibetan Rites

Other Works by Carolinda Witt

The Illustrated Five Tibetan Rites
The 10-Minute Rejuvenation Plan
Double Agent Celery MI5's Crooked Hero

THE EYE OF REVELATION

1939 & 1946 EDITIONS COMBINED
The True Five Tibetan Rites

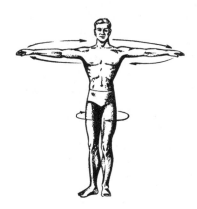

Peter Kelder &
Carolinda Witt

Includes

The Eye of Revelation (1939 and 1946 Editions)
by Peter Kelder

Additional practice information, tips, and advice
by Carolinda Witt
T5T Five Tibetan Rites Teacher
Founder and Developer of T5T®

THE EYE OF REVELATION
1939 & 1946 editions combined
The True Five Tibetan Rites

UnMind Pty Ltd
PO Box 818
NSW 2107
Australia

www.T5T.com

Paperback ISBN: 978-0-9870703-7-1
EBook ISBN: 978-0-9870703-6-4

Copy Design: Damonza
Interior Design: Lazar Kackarovski

Year of publication: 2010

To all those who practice The Five Tibetan Rites

TABLE OF
CONTENTS

FOREWORD BY THE ORIGINAL PUBLISHERS

*T*he *Eye of Revelation* is truly a revelation. It reveals to you information which has been known and used by men in far-distant lands for more than 25 centuries, but which is now available to you for the first time. It is information which has been thoroughly tried and tested. Information that will stem the tide of premature old age with its attendant weaknesses and senility. This is information for which Ponce de Leon, and thousands of others down through the ages, would have given all they possessed.

The Eye of Revelation will often produce remarkable mental and physical changes within a month. So much so, in fact, that one gains new hope and enthusiasm, with which to carry on. However, the greatest results come after the tenth week. When you stop to consider that the average person has endured his afflictions from 20 to 30 years, to obtain gratifying results in such a short time as weeks sounds almost miraculous.

As long as you live and practice *The Eye of Revelation* you will get more and still more gratifying results.

Most Important: The information given in *The Eye of Revelation* was, for centuries, confined strictly to men. Now, to the surprise and delight of all concerned, it has been found that women, too, get equally beneficial and amazing results.

Now, man or woman, can go on to grand and glorious things, regardless of environment or circumstances.

Get started at once on the marvellous work of youthification, and may success, health, energy, power, vigor, virility, and life dog your footsteps forever.

INTRODUCTION

This book is the first time Peter Kelder's classic story, *The Eye of Revelation*, written in 1939, has been combined with his 1946 edition. Kelder made significant changes to his instructions on how to perform 'The Five Tibetan Rites' in his 1946 version and added two entirely new chapters, which you'll read about later.

The Eye of Revelation tells the story of a Westerner known only as 'Colonel Bradford,' who discovered a secret sect of monks living in a remote Tibetan monastery. Despite their advanced years, these monks were remarkably healthy and youthful. Bradford lived and studied with the monks for several years, where they taught him their secret to what some refer to as the 'fountain of youth.' Bradford brought this knowledge back to the West, where it became known as 'The Five Tibetan Rites of Rejuvenation' — a daily ritual of five yoga-like movements, a breathing technique, and some simple spiritual practices involving vocalized sound and mental techniques.

Since 1946, various versions of *The Eye of Revelation* have been and continue to be published. Some have been strongly edited to appeal to more current thinking and style, and others have introduced elements that did not exist in Peter Kelder's original works at all. For example, Kelder never used the word 'chakras,' referring to what he described as 'magnetic centers' as 'vortexes' only.

This book contains <u>Kelder's own words</u> and illustrations precisely as he created them long ago - reproduced here from the scans of rare 1939 & 1946 editions of *The Eye of Revelation*, owned by the late antiquarian book collector and seller Jerry Watt (RIP). I share Jerry's desire to keep the original words intact for future generations, which is why he gave me these scans with his full permission to publish them as I saw fit.

I have not changed Kelder's text at all, and some of you will notice punctuation and grammatical errors, which I have not corrected. This is intentional, as I believe it adds a greater sense of time and place to the story.

I have also shared some of what I have learned in my twenty-three years of teaching the Rites, including practice tips, insights, additional information, and suggestions on what to avoid when learning the Rites. I hope you will find it helpful.

Note

1. *The tips and information I have shared with you have been written in italics to distinguish them from the original.*

2. There isn't the space to include everything I have learned about the Rites in this book. So, if you require more in-depth information on how to practice the Rites, please check out my book, *The Illustrated Five Tibetan Rites* (263 photos & illustrations) or my Online Training Course with videos. (See the back of this book for details.)

1

THE BENEFITS OF THE FIVE TIBETAN RITES

The reasons why people learn and practice the Rites.
How about you – what are your reasons?

Attracted to the anti-aging benefits of the Rites.

Have noticed the first signs of aging and want to do whatever you can to stop-the-clock.

To increase your energy, mental agility and focus.

Want a simple, daily routine that improves motivation, mood and purpose.

To maintain a regular exercise routine, and adopt a healthier lifestyle.

Improve strength and flexibility.

Lead busy lives, and want a form of exercise that fits into your daily routine. Like the fact this routine takes just 10 to 15 minutes per day to practice once learned.

Strengthen your back to reduce back-ache or rehabilitate an injury (with doctor's approval.)

Like the idea of practicing yoga, but don't have the time or perhaps desire to attend classes.

Can be done anywhere, at any time. No special equipment or facilities needed.

The typical benefits people receive from doing the Rites vary from person to person. For some, the effects are dramatic, and for others, the improvements they notice at the beginning soon become part of their normal physiology. Others may not experience much of a change at all but describe a strong sense that the Rites are improving their health and vitality.

The cumulative benefits, however, do seem to continue, and there are many people in their 70s to 90s still doing the Rites after 20 or 30 years of practice.

Mention must be made here of exaggerated claims about the benefits of the Rites that have proliferated over the internet. This appears to have started when online marketers began selling a version of 'The Eye of Revelation' on a commission basis. They had no experience in teaching the Rites and may not have practiced them personally. Some certainly didn't, promoting the Rites as some kind of miracle cure.

People were led to believe that the Rites would completely halt their aging, help them lose enormous amounts of weight, and fix their cancer, heart disease, fibroid cysts, and numerous other serious health conditions. This diluted the Rites' credibility and increased people's expectations so high that disillusionment was inevitable. Anything short of a miracle was therefore seen as somewhat ho-hum.

In fact, the monks who developed the Rites didn't describe specific benefits – they simply stated that the specific purpose of the Rites is to regain health, youth, and vitality:

> "The body has seven centers, which, in English, could be called Vortexes. These are kind of magnetic centers. They revolve at great speed in the healthy body, but when slowed down – well, that is just another name for old age, ill-health, and senility. The quickest way to regain health, youth, and vitality is to start these magnetic centers

spinning again. There are but five practices that will do this. Any one of them will be helpful, but all five are required to get glowing results. These five exercises are really not exercises at all, in the physical culture sense. The Lamas think of them as 'Rites,' and so instead of calling them exercises or practices, we too shall call them 'Rites.'"

~ **Peter Kelder**, *The Eye of Revelation.*

THE POWER OF BELIEF

While it is important to have realistic expectations, the power of belief (or faith) is still a vital force. Colonel Bradford, the principal character of this story said you need to invest a strong amount of faith and belief in the Rites to maximize their benefit. If you think old, you behave old, for example. Standing up straight is one of the most potent ways of looking younger, and these Rites will help improve your posture to do so.

A good example of this is the medical use of placebos. A common practice is to give patients an inert sugar pill without telling them the pill is a placebo. Having been told the pill will improve their condition, the patient's belief does indeed have a therapeutic effect, improving the condition it was intended for.

SO, WHAT KIND OF BENEFITS CAN YOU EXPECT?

To produce this list, I have not relied on hearsay; I have compiled the information from the feedback forms of many hundreds of students who attended our Five Tibetan Rites workshops and the testimonials of those who learned the Rites from my books, online course, or DVD. The point being made here is that this list represents the range of benefits experienced by 'real' people.

A significant increase in energy – more the endurance type of energy as opposed to the revved-up caffeine type of energy. You feel like you can keep going and going.

Feel calmer and less stressed – your buttons simply don't get pushed as easily anymore.

Develop significant mental clarity with razor-sharp focus.

Feel stronger, more flexible, and less stiff.

Enjoy seeing muscles appear on your arms, stomachs, hips, legs, and backs. Good for toning flabby arms, and tightening the abdomen.

Sleep better. Some people have more vivid dreams.

Overall improvement in your health, don't seem to catch colds, etc., as often. Helps with depression and anxiety – lifts mood and improves well-being. More centered and at peace.

Improved self-discipline and sense of purpose.

Feel younger and more powerful.

Improved breathing – deeper, slower, and more conscious.

Increased levels of Qi (chi, prana, life-energy).

Better posture.

Develops good core strength, which provides a strong foundation for any other form of exercise or modern living.

Some people lose weight; most find it easier to control weight and desire healthier foods.

Improved digestion and elimination.

Helps with the transition and symptoms of menopause.

Helps with the symptoms of menstruation.

Improved libido.

Many people also claim the Rites have made significant improvements to their health conditions. You can read their testimonials on the T5T website.

HEALTH
CONSIDERATIONS

2

Whenever you begin a new exercise program, there are always health considerations to consider. The information in this section is by no means comprehensive, and you should not substitute it for the direct advice of your doctor or health care provider.

If you feel any unusual discomfort or pain when you begin the Rites, stop practicing the exercises immediately, and discuss the situation with your qualified healthcare provider. If you have had a previous injury or are suffering from one at the moment, you must check with your health practitioner to ensure that the Rites will not aggravate your injury. Also, if you have a history of knee, shoulder, back, or neck injuries, it is always advisable to consult a qualified medical professional before attempting any of the postures.

PREGNANCY

It's important to note that the Rites are not intended for pregnant women, as this is not the best time for you to begin a new workout program, particularly without the advice of a qualified health or fitness professional. If you are pregnant and have already been practicing yoga or Pilates regularly, you should discuss this program with a qualified prenatal yoga or Pilates Instructor, as modifications or alterations may be possible. However, some of *these exercises are not recommended, particularly in late-term. Once your baby is delivered, you'll find that the exercises are an excellent way to get yourself back into shape, and they can be done while the baby sleeps – or at a time that suits you.*

You should consult your physician before commencing the Rites if you have any of the following serious medical or psychological problems:

- *Heat valve problems*
- *Enlarged heart*
- *Recent heart attack*
- *High or low blood pressure*
- *Cancer*
- *Meniere's disease*
- *Vertigo*
- *Multiple sclerosis*
- *Parkinson's disease*
- *Seizure disorders*
- *Mental illness*

Also, consult your physician if you are taking drugs that cause dizziness, if you have had recent abdominal or chest surgery, or if you suffer from any of the following:

- *Hernia*
- *Ulcers*
- *Hyperthyroidism*
- *Chronic fatigue syndrome*
- *Disc disease*
- *Fibromyalgia*
- *Severe arthritis of the spine*

- *Carpal tunnel syndrome*
- *Lower back injury*
- *Retinal or eye pressure (glaucoma)*

3

COLONEL BRADFORD'S GREAT DISCOVERY – PART ONE

One afternoon I dropped into the Travelers Club to escape a sudden shower, and while seated in an easy chair I fell into conversation with a most interesting old gentleman; one who, although I did not know it then, was destined to change the whole course of my life. I call him an old man for that is exactly what he was. In his late sixties, he looked every year his age. He was thin and stooped, and when he walked leaned heavily on his cane.

It developed that he was a retired British army officer, who had seen service in the diplomatic corps of the Crown. There were few accessible places on the globe to which Colonel Bradford, as I shall call him, although that was not his true name, had not, at some time or other in his life, paid a visit. Warming under my attention he related incidents in his travels which were highly entertaining. Needless to say, I spent an interesting afternoon listening to him. This was some years ago. We met often after that and got along famously. Many evenings, either at his quarters or at mine, we discussed and discoursed until long past midnight.

It was on one of these occasions I became possessed of a feeling that Colonel Bradford wanted to tell me something of importance. Something close to his heart which was difficult for him to talk about. By using all the tact and diplomacy at my command I succeeded in making him understand that I should be happy to help him in any way possible, and that if he cared to tell me what was on his mind I would keep it in strict confidence. Slowly at first, and then with increased trust he began to talk.

While stationed in India some years ago, Colonel Bradford, from time to time, came in contact with wandering natives from the remote fastnesses of the country. He heard many interesting tales of the life and customs of the country. One story, which interested him strangely, he heard quite a number of times, and always from natives who inhabited a particular district. Those from other districts never seemed to have heard this story.

It concerned a group of Lamas or Tibetan priests who, apparently, had discovered "The Fountain of Youth." The natives told of old men who had mysteriously regained health and vigor, strength and virility shortly after entering a certain lamasery; but where this particular place was none seemed exactly to know.

Like so many other men, Colonel Bradford had become old at 40, and had not been getting any younger as the years rolled by. Now the more he heard this tale of "The Fountain of Youth" the more he became convinced that such a place and such men actually existed. He began to gather information on directions, character of the country, climate, and various other data that might help him locate the spot; for from then on there dwelt in the back of his mind a desire to find this "Fountain of Youth."

This desire, he told me, had now grown so powerful that he had determined to return to India and start in earnest a quest for the retreat of the young-old men; and he wanted me to go with him. Frankly, by the time he had finished telling me this fantastic story I, too, was convinced of its truth, and was half-tempted to join him, but I finally decided against it.

Soon he departed, and I consoled myself for not going with the thought that perhaps one should be satisfied to grow old gracefully; that perhaps the Colonel was wrong in trying to get more out of life than was vouchsafed to other men. And yet – a Fountain of Youth!!! What a thrilling idea it was! For his own sake I hoped that the old Colonel might find it.

Months passed. In the press of every-day affairs Colonel Bradford and his "Shangri-La" had grown dim in my memory, when one evening on returning to my apartment, there was a letter in the Colonel's own handwriting. He was still alive! The letter seemed to have been written in joyous desperation. In it he said that in spite of maddening delays and set-backs he actually was on the verge of finding the "Fountain." He gave no address.

It was more months before I heard from him again. This time he had good news. He had found the "Fountain of Youth"! Not only that, but he was bringing it back to the States with him, and would arrive within the next two months. Practically four years had elapsed since I had last seen the old man. Would he have changed any, I wondered? He was older, of course, but perhaps no balder, although his stoop might have increased a little. Then the startling idea came to me that perhaps this "Fountain of Youth" might really have helped him. But in my mind's eye I could not picture him differently than I had seen him last, except perhaps a little older.

One evening I decided to stay at home by myself and catch up on my reading, maybe write a few letters. I had finally settled down to comfortable reading when the telephone rang.

"A Colonel Bradford to see you, sir," said the desk clerk.

"Send him up," I shouted. In a short time a rap was heard on the door. I opened it in haste. For a moment I stared, and then with dismay I saw that this was not the Colonel Bradford I was hoping to see, but a much younger man.

Noting my surprise he said, "Weren't you expecting me?"

"No," I confessed. "I thought it would he an old friend of mine, a Colonel Bradford."

"I came to see you about Colonel Bradford, the man you were expecting," he answered.

"Come in," I invited.

"Allow me to introduce myself," said the stranger, entering. "My name is Bradford."

"Oh, you are Colonel Bradford's son," I exclaimed. "I have often heard him speak of you so often. You resemble him somewhat."

"No, I am not my son," he returned. "I am none other than your old friend, Colonel Bradford, the old man who went away to the Himalayas."

I stood in incredulous amazement at his statement. Then it slowly dawned upon me that this really was the Colonel Bradford whom I had known; but what a change had taken place in his appearance. Instead of the stooped, limping, sallow old gentleman with a cane, he was a tall, straight, ruddy-complexioned man in the prime of life.[1] Even his hair, which had grown back, held only a trace of grey.[2]

(1) *The Rites improve your posture by strengthening your back and abdominal muscles so you can hold yourself erect. Together with a conscious decision to remove 'old people mannerisms' from yourself, like stooping, slumping, dithering, etc., you'll feel more energetic, and people will say how much younger you look. You'll feel it too.*

(2)   *I don't want to disillusion anyone, but I have only once*
seen a mild change in hair color. The sideburns of one of my
students appeared to have darkened after several months
of practice. Going from completely grey to completely dark
is probably unrealistic, and if it happened regularly would
be reported on the front-page news!

My enthusiasm and curiosity knew no bounds. Soon I was plying him with questions in rapid-fire order until he threw up his hands.

"Wait, wait," he protested, laughingly. "I shall start at the beginning and tell you all that has happened." And this he proceeded to do.

Upon arriving in India the Colonel started directly for the district in which lived the natives who had told of "The Fountain of Youth." Fortunately, he knew quite a bit of their language. He spent a number of months there, making friends with the people and picking up all the information he could about the Lamasery he sought. It was a long, slow process, but his shrewdness and persistence finally brought him to the coveted place he had heard about so often, but only half-believed existed.

Colonel Bradford's account of what transpired after being admitted to the Lamasery sounded like a fairy tale. I only wish that time and space permitted me to set down here all of his experiences; the interesting practices of the Lamas, their culture, and their utter indifference to the work-a-day world. There were no real old men there. To his surprise the Lamas considered Colonel Bradford a quite novel sight, for it had been a long time since they had seen anyone who looked as old as he. The Lamas good-naturedly referred to the Colonel as "The Ancient One."

"For the first two weeks after I arrived," said the Colonel, "I was like a fish out of water. I marvelled at everything I saw, and at times could hardly believe what my eyes beheld. I soon felt much better, was sleeping like a top every night, and only used my cane when hiking in the mountains.

"About three months after I arrived I received the biggest surprise of my life. In fact, I was quite startled. It was the day I entered for the first time, a large, well-ordered room which was used as a kind of library for ancient manuscripts. At one end of the room was a full-length mirror. It had been over two years since I had last seen my reflection, so with great curiosity I stepped in front of the glass.

"I stared in amazement, so changed was my appearance. It seemed that I had dropped 15 years from my age. It was my first intimation that I was growing younger; but from then on I changed so rapidly that it was apparent to all who knew me.

Soon the honorary title of "The Ancient One" was heard no more."

A knock at the door interrupted the Colonel. I opened it to admit a couple of friends from out of town who had picked this most inauspicious time to spend a sociable evening with me. I hid my disappointment and chagrin as best I could and introduced them to Colonel Bradford. We all chatted together for a short time, and then the Colonel said, as he arose:

"I am sorry that I must leave so early, but I have an appointment with an old friend who is leaving the city tonight. I hope I shall see you all again shortly."

At the door he turned to me and said, softly, "Could you have lunch with me tomorrow? I promise, if you can do so, you shall hear all about 'The Fountain of Youth.'"

We agreed as to the time and place and the Colonel departed. As I returned to the living room, one of my friends remarked,

"That is certainly a most interesting man, but he looks awfully young to be retired from Army service."

"How old do you suppose he is?" I asked.

"Well, he doesn't look forty," answered my friend, "but from the experiences he has had I suppose he must be that old."

"Yes, he's all of that," I replied evasively, and deftly turned the conversation into another channel. I thought it best to arouse no wonderment regarding the Colonel until I knew what his plans were.

The next day, after having lunch together, we repaired to the Colonel's room in a nearby hotel, and there at last he told me about "The Fountain of Youth."

"The first important thing I was taught after entering the Lamasery," he began, "was this. The body has seven centers which, in English, could be called Vortexes. These are kind of magnetic centers. They revolve at great speed in the healthy body, but when slowed down – well, that is just another name for old age, ill-health, and senility.

"There are two of these Vortexes in the brain; one at the base of the throat; another in the right side of the body opposite the liver; one in the sexual center; and one in each knee.

"These spinning centers of activity extend beyond the flesh in the healthy individual, but in the old, weak, senile person they hardly reach the surface, except in the knees. The quickest way to regain health, youth, and vitality is to start these magnetic centers spinning again.

"There are but five practices that will do this. Any one of them, especially the first, will be helpful, but all five are usually required to get glowing results. These five exercises are really not exercises at all, in the physical culture sense. The Lamas think of them as 'Rites,' and so instead of calling them exercises or practices, we too, shall call them Rites."

THERE ARE SEVEN PSYCHIC VORTEXES IN THE PHYSICAL BODY

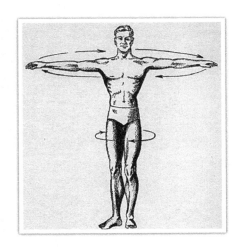

There are SEVEN Psychic Vortexes in the physical body. Vortex "A" is located within the forehead; Vortex "B" is located in the posterior part of the brain; Vortex "C" is located in the right side of the body above the waist line; Vortex "E" is located in the reproductive anatomy, **and it is directly connected with Vortex "C" in the throat**. Vortexes "F" and "G" are located in either knee.

The text in bold above was not included in the 1946 update.

- **Vortex "A"** is located **deep** within the forehead.
- **Vortex "B"** is in the posterior part of the brain.
- **Vortex "C"** located in throat at the base of the neck.
- **Vortex "D"** located in the right side of the body (waist line).
- **Vortex "E"** is in the reproductive anatomy or organs, **and it is directly connected with Vortex "C" in the throat.**
- **Vortexes "F"** and **"G"** located one in either knee.

The text in bold above for Vortexes "A" and "E" were added to the 1946 update.

These Psychic Vortexes revolve at great speed. When all are revolving at the same speed the body is in good health. When one or more of them slow down, old age, loss of power, or senility begin to set in almost immediately.

THE FIVE TIBETAN RITES ON ONE PAGE

*Most people find it helpful to have the full sequence from 1-5 on one page – see images below. You can **also download and print** these posters for free on the T5T.com website (T5T is short for The Five Tibetans.)*

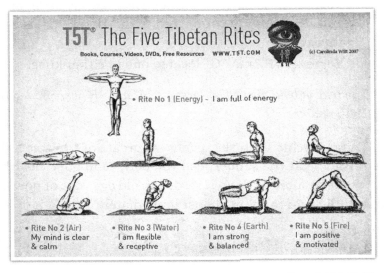

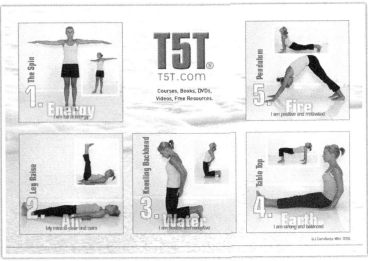

COMPARISONS BETWEEN THE ORIGINAL 1939 EDITION AND THE 1946 UPDATE

I have carefully compared the original 1939 version of 'The Eye of Revelation' to Peter Kelder's 1946 update in great detail. Surprisingly, Kelder didn't change the text's main body, but he did add two new chapters: "Mantram-Mind Magic" and "The Magic Quality of AUM."

Other than minor word replacements, Kelder's most significant changes were to his instructions on performing Rites No 1-5. In the initial 1939 version, there were no instructions beneath the images for each Rite - whereas in the 1946 version, Kelder has added new information. I have highlighted these changes in bold so you can compare them.

1. **1939 Edition:** *Kelder provides one or two illustrations and a story about each Rite. His descriptions are very brief, with just a few lines describing how one should do each movement.*

2. **1946 Edition:** *Using the space beneath the same images as in the 1939 version, Kelder added additional instructions and some amendments.*

3. *I have used **bold** to highlight these changes so you know what Kelder considered important enough to change.*

4. *I have not highlighted the few minor word changes he made, such as replacing the word "direction" with the word "way."*

BUILDING REPETITIONS

"To start with," said he, "I would suggest you practice each Rite three times a day for the first week. Then increase them by two a day each week until you are doing 21 a day, which will be at the beginning of the 10th week."

~ **Colonel Bradford** in *The Eye of Revelation*.

I recommend you follow Bradford's instructions to build up repetitions as he describes above. Many changes occur in the body, and it takes time to adjust. You can feel unbalanced, not present, scattered or moody when you do too many repetitions too quickly.

Some people are very keen to reach 21 repetitions as quickly as possible, but I can assure you that most of the gifts happen during the journey. Remember to enjoy the journey – your achievement will be more rewarding if you do so.

RITE
NUMBER ONE

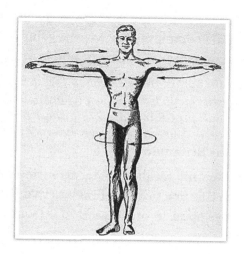

"The first Rite," continued the Colonel "is a simple one. It is for the express purpose of speeding up the Vortexes. When we were children we used it in our play. It is this:

Stand erect with arms outstretched, horizontal with the shoulders. Now spin around until you become slightly dizzy. There is only one caution: you must turn from left to right. In other words, if you were to place a clock or watch on the floor face up, you would turn in the same way the hands are moving. (*1939 & 1946 Editions*)

"At first the average adult will only be able to "spin around" about a half-dozen times until he becomes dizzy enough to want to sit or lie down. That is just what he should do, too. That's what I did. To begin with, practice this Rite only to the point of slight dizziness.[3] As time passes and your Vortexes become more rapid in movement through this and other Rites, you will be able to practice it to a greater extent.

"When I was in India it amazed me to see the *Maulawiyah*, or as they are more commonly known, the Whirling Dervishes, almost unceasingly spin around and around in a religious frenzy.

> (*Mawlawiyah, Turkish Mevleviyah, a fraternity of Sufis (Muslim mystics) founded in Konya (Qonya), Anatolia, by the Persian Sufi poet Rūmī (d. 1273), whose popular title mawlānā (Arabic: "our master") gave the order its name.*) –
> **Encyclopedia Britannica**

"Rite Number One recalled to my attention two things in connection with this practice. The first was that these Whirling Dervishes always spun in one direction – from left to right, or clockwise.

> *In fact, the Dervishes* **spin counterclockwise***, not clockwise, as described by Kelder above. Rumi's family describe the spin direction of the Dervishes during the "Sema," a religious ceremony carried out in remembrance of God below.*

"Revolving around the heart, from right to left, he embraces all the mankind, all the creation with affection and love."

~ Rumi's family – Mevlana.net

"The second was the virility of the old men; they were strong, hearty, and robust. Far more than most Englishmen are at their age.

"When I spoke to one of the Lamas about this, he informed me that while this whirling movement of the Dervishes did have a very beneficial effect, yet it also had a devastating one. It seems that a long siege of whirling stimulates into great activity Vortexes "A," "B," and "E." These three have a stimulating effect on the other two– "C" and "D." But due to excessive leg action the Vortexes in the knees– "E" and "G" – are over-stimulated and finally so exhausted that the building up of the Vital Forces along with this tearing down causes the participants to experience a kind of "psychic jag" which they mistake for something very spiritual.

"However," continued the Colonel, "we do not carry the whirling exercise to excess. While the whirling Dervishes may spin around many hundreds of times, we find that greater benefit is obtained by restricting it to about a dozen or so times, or enough so that Rite Number One can stimulate all the Vortexes to action. After several months it can be increased to 20 revolutions. Later to 30, 40, and eventually, after many months, to 50."

(3) *If you experience dizziness, don't be disheartened as it usually improves over time. I have seen fit people, and those who practice yoga regularly (including teachers) take around six months to build up to 21 repetitions of the spin because of dizziness. By far, the vast majority of people have no trouble at all unless they try to do too many repetitions, too quickly.*

The symptoms of dizziness/motion sickness occur because your brain receives conflicting information from your sensory systems. These senses send information to your brain about the position and movement of your body. This includes your eyes, the sensors of the semicircular canals in your inner ears, and the somatosensory receptors in your skin, joints, and muscles. A mismatch in sensory information causes a conflict between what is seen or felt and your previous orientational experience. When this happens, the body responds with the symptoms of dizziness and motion sickness. For this reason, using the correct technique during the spin is crucial.

*To reduce dizziness, try fine-tuning your movements by using the techniques described in **Appendix (A)**, on page 116.*

ALTERNATIVE TO THE SPIN

In the rare likelihood that dizziness becomes a problem for you – try this alternative.

> Simply swing your arms at shoulder height around to the opposite shoulder, and repeat to the other side. Your head and upper body twist around to one side and then the other. Your feet remain stationary, but remember to lift the opposite heel to the direction you are turning to avoid straining your lower back.

There is no twisting movement in The Five Tibetan Rites, so this exercise improves flexibility and reduces tension. I do it every day because it feels so good.

RITE
NUMBER TWO

"Like Rite Number One," continued the Colonel, "this second one is for further stimulating to action the Seven Vortexes. It is even simpler than the first one. In Rite Number Two, one first lies flat on his back on the floor or on the bed.[4] If practiced on the floor, one should use a rug or blanket under him, folded several times in order that the body will not come into contact with the cold floor.

The Lamas have what in English might be called a 'prayer rug.' It is about two feet wide and fully six feet long. It is fairly thick and is made from wool and a kind of vegetable fibre. It is solely for the purpose of insulation, and so has no other value. Nevertheless, to the Lamas everything is of a religious nature, hence their name for these mats – 'prayer rugs.'

"As I said, one should lie full length on his 'prayer rug' or bed. Then place the hands flat down alongside the hips. The fingers should be kept close together with the fingertips of each hand turned slightly toward one another. The feet are then raised until the legs are straight up. If possible, let the feet extend back a bit over the body, toward the head; but do not let the knees bend. Then, slowly lower the feet to the floor and for a moment allow all muscles to relax. Then perform this Rite all over again.

"One of the Lamas told me that when he first attempted to practice this simple Rite he was so old, weak, and decrepit that he couldn't possibly lift up both legs. Therefore he started out by lifting the thighs until the knees were straight up, letting the feet hang down. Little by little, however, he was able to straighten out his legs until eventually he could raise them straight with perfect ease.

"I marveled at this particular Lama," said the Colonel, "when he told me this. He was then a perfect picture of health and youth, although I knew he was many years older than he looked.

For the sheer joy of exerting himself, he used to carry up a pack of vegetables weighing fully a hundred pounds on his back, from the garden to the Lamasery, several hundred feet above. He took his time but never stopped once on the way up, and when he would arrive he didn't seem to be experiencing the slightest bit of fatigue. I marveled greatly at this, for the first time I started up with him, and I was carrying no load, I had to stop at least a dozen times. Later I was able to do it easily without my cane and with never a stop."

(4)   *Avoid practicing the Leg Raise on your bed unless your bed is very firm. Soft and padded mattresses are generally a modern development, and any sagging in the mattress caused by your body weight changes your spine's natural and optimal S-shape, creating additional strain on the supporting muscles that protect your pelvis, neck, and spine. Since these movements are done repetitively, you should do Rite No 2 on the floor, using a yoga mat, rug, or carpet for comfort.*

RITE NO 2 – THE LEG RAISE

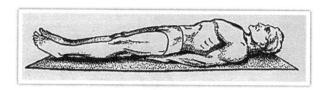

First Position of Rite No. 2

"One should lie full length on his 'prayer-rug,' or bed. Then place the hands flat alongside the hips. Fingers should be kept close together with the finger-tips [*sic*] of each hand turned slightly toward one another." (*1939 & 1946 Editions – Introduction.*)

To perform this Rite lie full length on rug or bed. Place the hands **flat down** alongside of the hips. Fingers should be kept close together with the finger-tips of each hand turned slightly toward one another. (*1946 Edition – beneath the image.*)

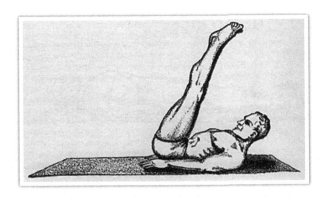

Second Position of Rite No. 2

The feet are then raised until the legs are straight up. If possible, let the feet extend back a bit over the body, toward the head ; but do not let the knees bend. Then, slowly lower the feet to the floor and for a moment allow all muscles to relax. Then perform this Rite all over again. (*1939 & 1946 Editions – Introduction.*)

"Raise the feet until the legs are straight up. If possible, let the feet extend back a bit over the body toward the head, but do not let the knees bend.[5] **Hold this position for a moment or two** and then slowly lower the feet to the floor, and for the **next several** moments allow all of the muscles **in the body to relax completely**. Then perform this Rite all over again.

While the feet and legs are being raised it is a good idea also to raise the head, then while the feet and legs are being lowered to the floor lower the head at the same time.

By raising the head at the same time the legs and feet are raised, all of the Vortexes in the body are

increased in their speed or action, but especially the slow ones." (*1946 Edition – beneath the image.*)

(5) *If you have suffered back pain in the past or are unfit, I recommend you avoid bringing your legs back over the stomach, as illustrated above, as it takes the spine out of its natural 'neutral' position. Neutral spine is a term used to describe the natural S-shape of the spine when its natural curves are maintained. The muscles closest to the spine (the core muscles) are more effective at stabilizing and protecting the spine (like guide wires on a tent) when the spine is in neutral.*

When you bring your legs back over your stomach, as illustrated above, your tailbone lifts, and the curve of your lower back is flattened to the floor. Instead, only raise your legs to a point where your knee bones are aligned over your hip bones (joint over joint), and the natural curve of your lower back remains intact. It makes no difference to the benefits of the Rites if you don't bring your legs back over your stomach.

If you need to bend your knees initially and then gradually straighten them as your flexibility increases, this is preferable to straining your lower back or neck.

7

RITE
NUMBER THREE

" The third Rite should be practiced immediately after practicing Rite Number Two. It, too, is a very simple one. All one needs to do is to kneel on his 'prayer rug,' place his hands on his thighs, and lean forward as far as possible with the head inclined so that the chin rests on the chest. Now lean backward as far as possible; at the same time the head should be lifted and thrown back as far as it will go. Then bring the head up along with the body. Lean forward again and start the rite all over. This Rite is very effective in speeding up Vortexes 'E,' 'D,' and 'C'; especially 'E.'

"I have seen more than 200 Lamas perform this Rite together. In order to turn their attention within, they closed their eyes. In this way they would not become confused by what others were doing and thus have their attention diverted.

"The Lamas, millenniums ago, discovered that all good things come from within. They discovered that <u>every worthwhile thing has its origin within the individual</u>. This is something that the Occidental has never been able to understand and comprehend. He thinks, as I did, that all worthwhile things must come from the outside world.

"The Lamas, especially those at this particular Lamasery, are performing a great work for the world. It is performed, however, on the astral plane. This plane, from which they assist mankind in all quarters of the globe, is high enough above the vibrations of the world to be a powerful focal point where much can be accomplished with little loss of effort."

"Someday the world will awaken in amazement to what the unseen forces – the Forces of Good – have been doing for the masses. We who take ourselves in hand and make new creatures of ourselves in every imaginable way, each is doing a marvelous work for mankind everywhere. Already the efforts of these advanced individuals are being welded together into One Irresistible Power. It is only through individuals like the Lamas, and you and me, that the world can possibly be helped.

"Most of mankind, and that includes those in the most enlightened countries, like America, Canada and England, is still in the darkest of the Dark Ages. However, they are being prepared for better and more glorious things, and as fast as they can be initiated into the higher life, just that fast will the world be made a better place in which to live."

RITE NO 3 – THE KNEELING BACKBEND

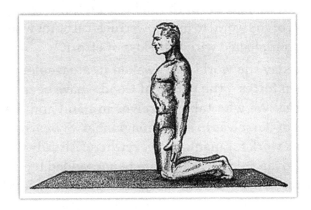

First Position of Rite No. 3

"All one needs to do is kneel on his 'prayer rug,' place his hands on his thighs, and lean forward as far as possible with the head inclined so that the chin rests on the chest." (*1939 & 1946 Editions – Introduction.*)

"The first position of this Rite is to kneel on a rug or mat **with hands at sides, palms flat against the side of the legs.** Then lean forward as far as possible,[6] **bending at the waist, with head well forward – chin on chest.**" (*1946 Edition – beneath the image.*)

(6)   *Check out the differences between the 1939 and 1946 descriptions highlighted in bold above. You will see that the illustration for the first part of Rite No 3 does not depict any bending at the waist, as described by Kelder. This causes confusion, so what should you do?*

   I recommend you learn and practice Rite No 3 without the forward bending action until your strength and flexibility increase. Once you have done so, you can experiment with the forward-bending, which doesn't appear to have any additional benefits over and above what you already receive from this Rite – at least not one you can detect.

Ideally, it is best for anyone doing this Rite to keep their spine 'long and strong' and to avoid collapsing in the lower back or neck during the movement, regardless of whether they do the forward bending movement or not. Repeatedly overbending in the lower back and neck compresses the vertebrae and discs, which can lead to strain and injury in vulnerable people—notably, older, unfit, or overweight people and anyone who has previously suffered back or neck pain.

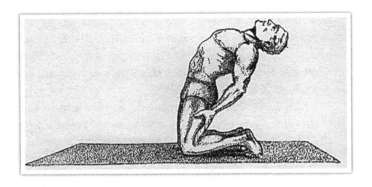

Second Position of Rite No. 3

"Now lean backward as far as possible; at the same time the head should be lifted and thrown back as far as it will go.[7] Then bring the head up along with the body. Lean forward again and start the rite all over. This Rite is very effective in speeding up Vortexes, 'E,' 'D,' and 'C'; especially 'E.'" (*1939 & 1946 Editions – Introduction.*)

> "The second position of this Rite is to lean backward as far as possible.[8] **Cause the head to move still further backward. The toes will prevent you from falling over backward.**
>
> **The hands are always kept against the side of the legs. Next come to an erect (kneeling) position, relax as much as possible for a moment,** and perform Rite all over again." (*1946 Edition – beneath the image.*)

(7) *If you feel dizzy or faint during this movement, avoid dropping your head back "as far as it will go," as this compresses the vertebrae and discs in your neck and may occlude (kink) the vertebral artery, temporarily reducing*

oxygen supply to your brain. Instead, keep your neck long and strong, and don't let your head drop back so far.

(8) As you can imagine, "*leaning as far back as possible*" creates a significant load on the lower back muscles to perform the movement and counter the effects of gravity at the same time.

Some people lean back on their thighs to give the appearance of a deeper arch, but with repetition, the thigh and groin muscles can become strained.

Instead, keep your hip bones aligned over your knee bones and your breastbone lengthened upwards (without puffing out your ribs) as described in Step 1, as you return to the starting position. Don't collapse; maintain the length of your spine as you return to the forward starting position.

Initially, you may feel this way of doing Rite 3 is less strenuous, but this is deceptive. Try squeezing your shoulder blades together at the back as you arch backward to increase the stretch. In our daily forward-facing actions, the muscles in our shoulders and chest become stiff as very few natural movements cause us to lean backward. Take advantage of the backbend to stretch and loosen these muscles to relieve tension and increase mobility. It feels good too.

8

RITE
NUMBER FOUR

"Now for Rite Number Four," said the Colonel. "The first time I tried this it seemed very difficult, but after a while it was as simple to do as any of the others.[9]

"Sit on the 'prayer rug' with the feet stretched out in front. Then place the hands alongside the body. Now raise the body and bend the knees so that the legs, from the knees down, are practically straight up and down. The arms, too, will be straight up and down, while the body, from the shoulders to the knees, will be horizontal. Before pushing the body to a horizontal position, the chin should be well down on the chest. Then, as the body is raised, the head should be allowed to drop gently backward as far as it will go. Next, return to a sitting position and relax for a moment before repeating the procedure. When the body is pressed up to the complete horizontal position, tense every muscle in the body. This will have a tendency to stimulate Vortexes 'F,' 'G,' 'E,' 'D' and C.'

"After leaving the Lamasery," continued Colonel Bradford, "I went to a number of the larger cities in India, and as an experiment conducted classes for both English people and natives. I found that the older members of either felt that unless they could perform a Rite perfectly, right from the beginning, they believed no good could come from it. I had considerable difficulty in convincing them that they were wrong. But after a good deal of persuasion I was able to get them to do their best, and the results were more than gratifying.

"I remember in one city I had quite a number of old people in one of my classes. With this particular Rite – Number Four – they could just barely get their bodies off the floor; they couldn't get it anywhere near a horizontal position. In the same class were several much younger persons who had no difficulty in performing the Rite perfectly from the very start. This so discouraged the older people that I had to ask the younger ones to refrain from practicing it before their older classmates.

I explained that I could not do it at first, either; that I couldn't do a bit better than any of them; but that I could perform the Rite 50 times in succession now without feeling the slightest strain on nerves or muscles; and in order to convince them, I did it right before their eyes. From then on, the class broke all records for results accomplished."

(9) *If you haven't got sufficient arm strength in the beginning, don't worry – try propping your hands on yoga blocks or folded towels (nothing slippery or uneven like cushions). It will make it easier to lift into the tabletop position. Then, as your arm strength increases, you can cut them in half to reduce the height or remove them altogether.*

RITE NO 4 – THE TABLETOP

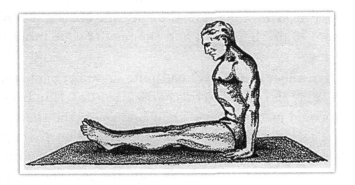

First Position of Rite No. 4

"Sit on the 'prayer rug' with the feet stretched out in front. Then place the hands alongside the body." (*1939 & 1946 Editions – Introduction.*)

"Sit **erect** on **rug or carpet** with feet stretched out in front. **The legs must be perfectly straight – back of knees must be well down or close to the rug. Place the hands flat on the rug, fingers together, and the hands pointing outward slightly. Chin should be on chest – head forward.**" (*1946 Edition – beneath the image.*)

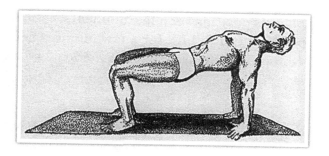

Second Position of Rite No. 4

"Now raise the body and bend the knees so that the legs from the knees down, are practically straight up and down. The arms, too, will be straight up and down while the body, from the shoulders to the knees, will be horizontal. Before pushing the body to a horizontal position the chin should be well down on the chest.

Then, as the body is raised the head should be allowed to drop gently backward as far as it will go.[10] Next, return to a sitting position and relax for a moment before repeating the procedure. When the body is pressed up to the complete horizontal position tense every muscle in the body.[11] This will have the tendency to stimulate Vortexes 'F,' 'G,' 'E,' 'D,' and 'C.'" (*1939 & 1946 Editions – Introduction.*)

"Now **gently** raise the body, **at the same time** bend the knees so that the legs from the knees down, are practically straight up and down. The arms, too, **will also be vertical** while the body from shoulders to knees will be horizontal.

As the body is raised **upward** allow the head gently to **fall** backward so that the head hangs backward as far as possible **when the body is fully horizontal.**

Hold this position for a few moments, return to first position and RELAX for a few minutes before performing the Rite again." (*1946 Edition – beneath the image.*)

(10) *For the same reasons as those mentioned in Rite No 3, avoid letting the head "drop gently backward as far as it will go" to prevent compression of your cervical spine and vertebral artery. Instead, keep your head balanced on top of your neck as if you were standing upright.*

(11) **Tensing All The Muscles.** *In his new instructions added beneath each illustration in his 1946 update, Kelder left out the sentence, "When the body is pressed up to the complete horizontal position tense every muscle in the body.'*

I mention this because some practitioners believe tensing is significant and perhaps mysterious. But, as you can see from the above, Kelder doesn't attach as much importance to it as they do. Another example of this is Kelder's inconsistency when describing tensing across each Rite. He doesn't mention tensing at all in Rites 2 and 3, and in Rite 4, he describes the effects of tensing on stimulating the vortexes but doesn't do the same for Rite No 5.

Perhaps Bradford simply means that when we reach the apex of the movement, all our muscles are tensed (which they are) before we move down into the second part of the movement. In practice, it is impossible to avoid having tension in your muscles at these two points in the movement due to the opposing forces of gravity.

Note: If you suffer from high blood pressure, avoid holding your breath when muscle tensing, as this can raise blood pressure.

RITE
NUMBER FIVE

9

"The best way to perform this Rite is to place the hands on the floor about two feet apart. Then, with the legs stretched out to the rear with the feet also about two feet apart, push the body, and especially the hips, up as far as possible, rising on the toes and hands. At the same time the head should be brought so far down that the chin comes up against the chest.

"After a few weeks, that is after you become quite proficient in this movement, let the body drop from its highest position to a point almost but not quite touching the floor. The muscles should be tensed for a moment when the body is at the highest point, and again at the lowest point. **Before the end of the first week this particular Rite will be one of the easiest ones to perform for the average person.**" *(1939 Edition. The sentence in bold above was not included in the 1946 update.)*

"The Second position is attained by pushing the body, especially the hips, upward as far as possible. The hands are kept flat on the floor at all times. Hold this position for a brief moment and return to First position. After a moment of "hanging in suspension" perform the Rite over again.

"Next, allow the body to come slowly down to a 'sagging' position. Bring the head up, causing it to be drawn as far back as possible.

"Everywhere I go," went on the Colonel, "folks, at first, call these Rites physical culture exercises. I would like to make it clearly understood that these are not physical culture exercises at all. They are only performed a few times a day; so few times that they could not possibly be of any value as physical culture movements. What the Rites actually do is this: They start the seven Vortexes spinning at a normal rate of speed; at the speed which is normal for, say, a young, robust, strong, virile man of twenty-five years of age.

"Now in such a person the Vortexes are all spinning normally at the same rate of speed. On the other hand, if you could view the seven Vortexes of the average middle-aged man – weak, unhealthy, and semi-virile, as he is – you would notice at once that some of the Vortexes had greatly slowed down in their spinning movement; and worse still, all were spinning at a different rate of speed – none of them working together in harmony. The slower ones allowed that part of the body which they govern to degenerate, deteriorate, and become diseased.

"The only INNER difference between youth and senility is simply the difference in the rate of speed at which the Vortexes are spinning. Normalize the different speeds, and the old man becomes a new man again."

RITE NO 5– THE PENDULUM

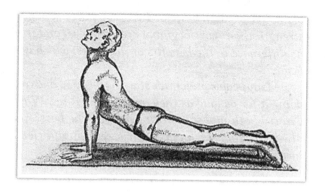

First Position of Rite No. 5

"The best way to perform this Rite[12] is to place the hands on the floor about two feet apart. Then, with the legs stretched out to the rear with the feet also about two feet apart, push the body, and especially the hips, up as far as possible, rising on the toes and hands. At the same time the head should be brought so far down that the chin comes up against the chest.

"Next, allow the body to come slowly down to a 'sagging' position. Bring the head up, causing it to be drawn as far back as possible. (*1939 & 1946 Editions – Introduction.*)

"The First position of the Rite is to place the hands on the floor about two feet apart. The legs are stretched out to the rear with the feet also about two feet apart. Allow the body to "sag"[13] **downward from shoulders to toes.** Hold the head as far back as is comfortable. **The arms are kept perfectly straight at all times in Rite No. 5.**" (*1946 Edition – beneath the image.*)

(12) When I began teaching the Rites, I experimented with starting this movement in the upside-down V position. The plank-like position described above requires more physical strength than most beginners can achieve, and it makes no difference to the benefits of this Rites, which way you begin.

Many people prefer this starting position and continue doing it for as long as they practice the Rites. Why don't you try both and see which suits you the best? You can always change back once your strength and flexibility increase.

(13) For the reasons discussed in Rite No 3, avoid 'sagging' in the lower back, as collapsing compresses your vertebrae and discs. Unless you know how to activate your core muscles correctly while maintaining the length in your spine, it is best to avoid overbending. Try gently firming your buttocks instead to prevent you from hollowing out your lower back too much. In the early stages, some people rest their thighs on a bolster for the same reason.

If you want to learn how to identify and engage your core muscles correctly, consider a few Pilates classes or learn from one of the T5T resources listed at the back of this book.

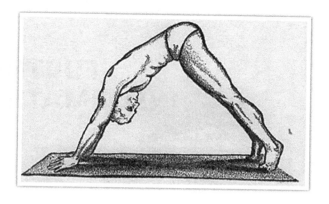

Second Position of Rite No. 5

"After a few weeks, that is after you become quite proficient in this movement, let the body drop from its highest position to a point almost but not quite touching the floor. The muscles should be tensed for a moment when the body is at the highest point, and again at the lowest point." (*1939 & 1946 Editions – Introduction.*)

"The Second position is attained by pushing the body, especially the hips, upward as far as possible. The hands are kept flat on the floor at all times. Hold this position for a brief moment and return to First position. After a moment of "hanging in suspension" perform the Rite over again. (*1946 Edition – beneath the image.*)

Note: As you can see, this entire description is new and is Kelder's biggest edit so far. It is also significant in that, once again, he doesn't mention muscle tensing– he merely says, "Hold this position for a brief moment."

10

FURTHER INFORMATION

W hen the Colonel had finished his description of the Five Rites I stopped him a moment.

"Let me ask you some questions now."

"Very well," he replied. "That is just what I want you to do."

"I feel that from your description I understand the Rites quite well," I began, "but when and how often are they to be employed?"

"They can be used either night and morning," answered the Colonel, "in the morning only, or just at night, if it is more convenient. I use them both morning and night, but I would not advise so much stimulation for the beginner until he has practiced them for a number of months. At the start he could use them the full number of times in the morning, and then in the evening he could gradually build up until finally he is doing the same amount of practice as in the morning."

"Just how many times a day should a person use these Rites?" was my next question.

"To start with," said he, "I would suggest you practice each Rite three times a day for the first week. Then increase them by two a day each week until you are doing 21 a day; which will be at the beginning of the 10th week.[14]

(14) *Everyone wants to reach the goal of 21 repetitions – some as quickly as possible. However, there is a lot to be gained by building up repetitions exactly as described by Kelder (3 reps in your first week, adding 2 per week until you are doing 21 in ten weeks' time.) We humans are always rushing towards some future experience, and you would benefit significantly from slowing down and being present to your experiences when learning the Rites. Arriving at your destination of 21 repetitions will be all the more fulfilling if you do so.*

People who practice yoga regularly or keep themselves fit may want to progress at a much faster rate than Colonel Bradford recommends. This is understandable, but please remember that these exercises are designed to have a stimulating effect on the energy systems of your body. If, after having performed the Rites, you find it difficult to relax or remain focused; are moodier than usual; have difficulty sleeping, or feel you are "not in" your body – then reduce repetitions and build up more gradually.

If you feel slightly nauseous or have a mild headache, then you are doing too many repetitions – most likely due to the spinning movement of the 1st Rite. See Appendix (A), on page 116 for more information on dizziness.

DETOX EFFECTS

Due to the increased elimination of impurities and wastes and elevated oxygen levels in your body, you may experience some minor detox effects. Some people have strong changes, and others have none at all. If you do experience any of the following symptoms, they usually settle down within a week.

A metallic taste in the mouth.

Achy joints for a day or so.

Darker, stronger-smelling urine.

Diarrhoea or a strong bowel movement.

Initial constipation.

Slight nausea.

Initial fatigue as body balances itself.

Cold or flu-like symptoms that last a day.

A runny nose as sinuses clear.

A tic or involuntary muscle movement over one eye. A mild rash or pimples.

Moodiness, either a bit snappy or teary.

"If you cannot practice Rite Number One, the whirling one, the same number of times as the others, then do it only as many times as you can without getting too dizzy. The time will soon come, however, when you can practice it the full number of 21 times.

"If, for any reason, one or more of the Rites cannot be used at all, do not be discouraged; use the ones you can. Results will be a little slower, but that will be the only handicap.

"If one has been recently operated on for, say, appendicitis, or is afflicted with hernia, he should be very cautious in practicing Rites Numbers Two, Three, and Five. If one is very heavy, he should be cautious in the use of Number Five until his weight has been greatly reduced.

"All five of the Rites are of importance. Even though he may not be able to perform them the prescribed number of times the individual may rest assured that just a few times each day will be of benefit.

"I knew of one man who required more than a year before he could do it that many times. But he performed the other four without difficulty, gradually increasing the number until he was doing the full 21 on all four. He got very splendid results.

"Under certain conditions," added the Colonel, "there are some who find it difficult to perform Rite Number One at all, to begin with. But after having done the other four for about six months they are amazed at how easy it is to do Number One. Likewise with the other Rites. If for any reason one or more of them cannot be used, do not be discouraged; use what you can. Results, in that case, will be a little slower, but that is the only handicap.

"If one has been recently operated on for, say, appendicitis, or is afflicted with hernia, he should be very cautious in practicing Rites Number Two and Five. If one is very heavy, he should be cautious in the use of Number Five until his weight has been greatly reduced.

"All five of the Rites are of importance. Even though he may not be able to perform them the prescribed number of times, the individual may rest assured that just a few times each day will be of benefit.

"If, at the end of the fourth week, one finds that he cannot perform every one of the Rites the required number of times, he should note carefully the ones which he is forced to slight. Then, if he is performing the Five Rites in the morning, he should try to make up the deficiency in the evening. Or if he is performing the Rites in the evening, he should endeavor to find time in the morning to catch up.

In either event he should not neglect the other Rites, and *above all he should never strain himself.* If he goes about performing the Rites in an easy, interesting manner it will not be long before he finds everything working out satisfactorily, and that he is doing the Rites the required 21 times a day.

"Some people, acting on their own initiative, invent little aids for their practices. An old fellow in India found it impossible for him to perform Rite Number Four properly even once. He wouldn't be satisfied with just getting his body off the floor; he was determined that it should reach a horizontal position as the Rite prescribed. So he got a box about ten inches high and two and a half feet long. Upon this he put some bedding folded to the right size, and across this padded box he lay flat on his back. Then, with his feet on the floor at one end and his hands on the floor at the other he found it quite simple to raise his body to a horizontal position.

"Now while this little 'stunt' may not in itself have helped the old gentleman in performing the Rite the full 21 times, still the psychological effect of being able to raise his body as high as the much stronger men was undoubtedly quite stimulating and may have been quite beneficial. I do not particularly recommend this old man's aid, although it may help those who think it impossible to make progress in any other way; but if you have an inventive mind you will think of ways and means to help you in performing the more difficult Rites.

"These Rites are so powerful that if one were left out entirely while the other four were practiced regularly the full number of times, only the finest kind of results would be experienced. The First Rite alone will do wonders as evidenced by the Whirling Dervishes of whom we spoke. Had they spun around only a limited number of times, they would have found themselves greatly benefited, although they may not have attributed their improved condition to the whirling. The fact that they whirled from left to right and that the old men were virile and strong is ample proof that just this one Rite will have powerful effects.

"So if anyone finds that they simply cannot perform all five of these Rites, or that they cannot perform them all the full number of times, they may know that good results may still be experienced."

"Does anything else go with these Five Rites?" I asked.

"There is one more thing – just a suggestion. Take either a tepid bath or a cool, but not cold, one after practicing the Rites.

"Going over the body quickly with a wet towel and then with a dry one is probably even better. One thing I must caution you against: you must never take a shower, tub, or wet towel bath which is cold enough to chill you even slightly internally. If you do, you will have undone all the good you have gained from performing the Five Rites."

"This all seems so simple," I ventured, "Do you mean to tell me that this is all that is necessary in the work of restoring the prematurely old to robust health, vigor, and virility?"

"All that is required," answered the Colonel, "is to practice the Five Rites three times a day to begin with, and gradually increase them as I have explained until each is being practiced 21 times each day. That is all; there is nothing more.

"Of course," he continued, "one must practice them every day in order to keep one's robust vitality. You may skip one day a week, but never more than that. The use of the Five Rites is no hardship at all; it requires less than 10 minutes a day to practice them. If necessary one can get up ten minutes earlier or go to bed ten minutes later.

"The Five Rites are for the express purpose of restoring a man to manhood. That is, to make him virile and keep him that way constantly. Whether or not he will make the comeback in youthful appearance, as I have done in so short a time, depends on how he uses his virility.

"Some men do not care whether they look young, or even whether they appear young, just so long as they have all their manly powers. But as for me, I was an old man for so many years that I like the idea of throwing off the years in every way possible."

BREATHING

K elder gave NO instructions on how to breathe while practicing The Five Rites. It is only in later reprints by other publishers, including myself, that breathing methods are included with the Rites.

Apart from the 6th Rite, which is a breathing exercise, the only mention of breathing in the 1939 and the 1946 editions of "The Eye of Revelation" is to recommend that we **"stand erect with hands on hips between the Five Rites and take one or two deep breaths."**

Since correct respiration is vital to our overall health, energy, well-being, and longevity, I have added natural full breathing instructions and exercises to T5T. Many people have achieved enormous benefits from this.

Some people will object to anything being added to the Rites and believe they should remain exactly as described. If we did as they wished across all forms of comparable exercise, like yoga, physical fitness, Tai Chi, etc., our knowledge would not progress beyond what we knew seventy or 2,500 years ago (if the publishers claim about the age of the Rites is correct.)

I have therefore added full natural breathing to the Rites as it makes sense to include something as important as this to our daily wellness routine.

Breathing is so significant. It supplies life-giving energy (prana, chi) and oxygen to our bodies and removes wastes. A number of clinical studies have proven that how well you breathe literally dictates your lifespan.[15]

(15) **The Framingham study** These researchers were able to foretell how long a person was going to live by measuring forced exhalation breathing volume, FEV1, and hypertension. We know that much of hypertension is controlled by the way we breathe. "Long before a person becomes terminally ill, vital capacity can predict life span." William B. Kannel of Boston School of Medicine (1981)

"Life starts and stops with a breath. We survive without food for weeks, without water for days, but without air we cannot survive more than a few minutes. By taking control of our breathing and improving the way we breathe we will oxygenate our body more efficiently."

~ **Anders Olsson,** *Conscious Breathing*

Since Kelder didn't leave any breathing instructions other than "take one or two deep breaths" between each Rite –any form of breathing carried out with the Rites is entirely optional.

There are many breathing methods and teachers you can learn from, but if you wish to do as we at T5T have done for twenty-three years, please see the resources at the back of the book.

Our 'Energy Breathing' method, which we carry out between each Rite, is very popular, resulting in a calmer, more focused, and happier approach to life. We also breathe in a specific way while doing the Rites, which provides energy, balance, and stability to our movements.

If you would like to try the meditations based on breathing that we use in our workshops and online training course, you can download them on the T5T.com website for free.

12

THE FIVE ELEMENTS

A t the time of the development of the Five Tibetan Rites of Rejuvenation, the ancients believed that their world was composed of Five Elements: water, earth, air, fire, and spirit (energy).

In psychology, the Five Elements are used to personify different human traits, such as the personality type categories of Carl Jung (feeling, sensing, intuiting, and thinking) and those associated with the astrological signs of the zodiac. I experimented with the concept of adding an element and an affirmation to each of the Rites. Many people have found the results to be amazing. You can try them and see if they work as well for you.

In each case, the physical movement of the Rite was a metaphor for what we were trying to achieve mentally – awareness of a different aspect of life. For example, the Spin takes the element energy, and the vortex that the movements create allows you to replenish your body from the larger energy all around us. The Tabletop takes the element earth, and its movements focus on stability, foundation, and balance, giving us a solid base from which to form new ideas.

In holistic exercise, it can sometimes be hard to marry the physical state with the mental state, and having a metaphor helps people align the two and present a clear picture of what they are working towards.

Having assigned an element and a modern name to each Rite, I then experimented with creating an affirmation that expressed the "energy" of each movement. The result is a method of reinforcing and focusing on the positive benefits of each Rite physically, mentally, and spiritually. This has a ripple effect on every area of your life.

- **Rite No. 1 (Energy)**
  - *The Spin – "I am full of energy."*
- **Rite No. 2 (Air)**
  - *The Leg Raise – "My mind is clear and calm."*
- **Rite No. 3 (Water)**
  - *The Kneeling Backbend – "I am flexible and receptive."*
- **Rite No. 4 (Earth)**
  - *The Tabletop – "I am strong and balanced."*
- **Rite No. 5 (Fire)**
  - *The Pendulum – "I am positive and motivated."*

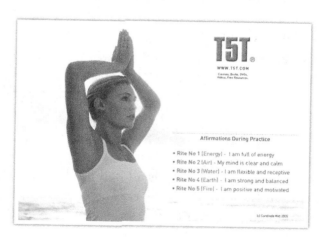

You can download this free *Affirmations Poster* on the T5T. com website.

13

THE HIMALAYA CLUB - PART TWO

I t had been ten weeks since Colonel Bradford's return from India. Much had happened in that time. I had immediately started putting the Five Rites into practice and had been getting results. The Colonel had been busy with some personal business transactions and I saw little of him for a while, but when he once more was at leisure I lost no time telling him of my progress and in enthusiastically expressing my feeling regarding this wonderful new system of regaining vigor, health, power, virility, and vitality.

Ever since the day I was sure that I was well on the way to -ment. The Colonel insisted that the class be limited to not more than 15 members, and I had ten times that number in mind. However, no amount of persuasion and coercion could change his mind.

From the beginning the class was a huge success. We met once a week and my friends all had implicit faith in the Colonel and in the Five Rites. As early as the second week I could see marked improvement in several of them, although, being forbidden to discuss their progress with anyone but the Colonel, I could not verify my impression. However, at the end of a month we held a kind of testimonial meeting. Every man reported improvement. Some told most glowing accounts. A man nearing 75 years of age had made more gains than any of the others.

The weekly meetings of "The Himalaya Club," as we had named it, continued. The tenth week rolled around and practically all of the members were performing all Five Rites 21 times a day. All of them were feeling better and some dropped a number of years from their appearance.

This brought to mind that several of them had asked the Colonel his age but that he had told them he would wait until the end of the tenth week to tell them. This was the evening, but as yet the Colonel had not put in an appearance. Someone suggested that each member write on a slip of paper what age he believed the Colonel to be and then they would compare notes. As the papers were being collected, in walked Colonel Bradford. He was told what had taken place.

"Bring them to me and I shall see how well you have estimated my age. Then I shall tell you what it really is."

The slips all read from 38 to 42. With great amusement the Colonel read them aloud.

"Gentlemen," he said, "I thank you. You are most complimentary. And as you have been honest with me, I shall be equally honest with you. I shall be 73 years of age on my next birthday."

The members stared in consternation and amazement. They found it hard to believe that one so youthful in appearance could have lived so long. Then they wanted to know why, inasmuch as they already felt half their former age, they, too, had not made more progress in youthful appearance.

"In the first place, gentlemen," the Colonel informed them, "you have only been doing this wonderful work for ten weeks. When you have been at it two years you will see a much more pronounced change. Then again, I have not told you all there is to know. I have given you Five Rites which are for the express purpose of restoring one to manly vigor and vitality.

"These Five Rites also make one appear more youthful; but if you really want to look and be young in every respect there is a Sixth Rite that you must practice. I have said nothing about it until now because it would have been useless to you without first having obtained good results from the other five."

The Colonel then informed them that in order to go further with the aid of this Sixth Rite it would be necessary for them to lead a more or less continent life.[16] He suggested that they take a week to think the matter over and decide whether or not they desired to do so for the rest of their lives. Then those who wished to go on would be given Rite Number Six. There were but five who came back the next week, although according to the Colonel this was a better showing than he had experienced with any of his classes in India.

(16) More or less 'continent' means more or less celibate (abstinence from sexual intercourse.)

When he had first told them about the Sixth Rite, the Colonel had made it clear that the procreative energy would be lifted up, and that this lifting-up process would cause not only the mind to be renewed but the entire body as well; but that it entailed certain restrictions with which the average man did not care to conform. Then he went on with this explanation.

Although no instructions are provided for women, many thousands of women worldwide have successfully practiced the Rites and obtained the same great benefits as men.

*It is important to acknowledge that the greatest percentage of practitioners, regardless of gender, only practice the **Five** Rites. As the many thousands of my students would testify,* *these five exercises are sufficient to obtain the great benefits described in this book.*

"In the average virile man," said the Colonel, "the life forces course downward, but in order to become a Superman they must be turned upward. This we call 'The Newer Use of the Reproductive Energy.' Turning these powerful forces upward is a very simple matter, yet man has attempted it in many ways for centuries and in almost every instance has failed. Whole religious orders in the Occidental World have tried this very thing, but they, too, have failed because they have tried to master the procreative energy by suppressing it. There is only one way to master this powerful urge, and that is not by dissipating or suppressing it but by TRANSMUTING it – transmuting it and at the same time lifting it upward. In this way you really and truly have discovered not only the 'Elixir of Life,' as the ancients called it, but you have put it to use as well, which is something the ancients were seldom able to do.

"Now this Rite Number Six is the simplest thing in the world to perform. It should only be practiced when one has an excess of procreative energy; when there is a definite desire for expression. It can be done so easily that it can be performed anywhere at any time. When one feels the powerful reproductive urge, here is all that is necessary:

"Stand erect and then let all the air out of the lungs, as one bends over and places his hands on his knees. Force out the last trace of air. Then, with empty lungs, stand erect, place hands on hips, and push down on them. This has a tendency to push up the shoulders. While doing this, pull in the abdomen just as far as possible, which raises the chest. Now hold this position as long as you can. Then when you are forced to take air into the empty lungs, let the air flow in through the nose. Exhale it through the mouth as you relax the arms and let them hang naturally at your sides. Then take several deep breaths through the mouth or nose and allow them to quickly escape through either the mouth or the nose. This constitutes one complete performance of Rite Number Six. About three are required to subdue the most powerful urge and to turn the powerful procreative or reproductive forces upward.

> *Interestingly, the Sixth Rite is similar to a yoga practice known as 'Uddiyana Bandha,' which means 'flying upward energy lock.' It is one of three bandhas (energy locks or valves) that are practiced together or individually at specific times during yoga postures, breathing, visualization, meditation, and other yogic practices.*
>
> *The bandhas direct energy (prana) throughout the body to release blockages and nourish corresponding areas. They bind or 'lock' the prana to prevent it from dissipating from the body. Bandhas, when released, allows the flow of kundalini energy up the central energy canal in the spinal column, which connects the base chakra to the crown chakra.*

"The only difference there is between the average virile man and the Superman is that the average lets the procreative urge flow downward while the Super-man turns the procreative urge upward and reproduces within himself a NEW MAN – a strong, powerful, magnetic man who is constantly growing younger, day by day, moment by moment. This is the true SUPER-MAN, who creates within himself the true 'ELIXIR OF LIFE.' Now you understand why it was unnecessary for me to have left my native England to find the 'Fountain of Youth'– it was within me all the time. Now you can see that when I wrote my friend here some time ago that I had found 'The Fountain of Youth' and was bringing it back with me, I meant just that. The Five Rites and the 'Fountain' are one.

"When I remember Ponce de Leon and his futile search for the 'Fountain' I think of how simple it would have been for him to stay at home and simply use it; but he, like myself, believed it was anywhere in the world except at home – within one's self.

"Please understand that in order to perform Rite Number Six it is absolutely necessary that a man have full masculine virility. He couldn't possibly raise up and transmute procreative energy if there were little or none to transmute. It is absolutely impossible for an impotent man or the one with little virility to perform this Rite. He shouldn't even attempt it, because it would only lead to discouragement, which might do him great harm. Instead he should first practice the other Five Rites until he has full masculine power, and this regardless of how young or how old he may be. Then when the first "full bloom of youth" is experienced within him, he may, then go on to the business of being a SUPER-MAN.

"The man of the world is interested only in the material things of the world, and for that reason should practice only the first five Rites until he feels the urge or desire within to become the SUPER-MAN. Then he should decide definitely; for a clean-cut start and a new life are absolutely necessary to those who lead the SUPER-LIFE. They are the ones who become MYSTICS, OCCULTISTS, and ADEPTS. They it is who truly see with THE EYE OF REVELATION.

"Again I say, let no man concern himself with the upturning of the sex currents until he is thoroughly satisfied in his own mind and heart that he truly desires to lead the life of the MYSTIC; then let him make the step forward, and success will crown his every effort.

14

RITE
NUMBER SIX

From my experience, people who are interested in practicing the Sixth Rite generally fall into two camps. The first will try it and see what happens, and the second will carry out further research, such as reading tantric texts or obtaining instruction from recognized tantric teachers.

According to author and scholar, Dr. Peter Baofu, "the tantric practitioner seeks to use the prana (divine power) that flows through the universe (including one's own body) to attain purposeful goals. These goals may be spiritual, material, or both. Most practitioners of tantra consider mystical experience imperative. Some versions of Tantra require the guidance of a guru."

In the process of working with energy, the tantric practitioner has various tools at hand: Yoga, visualizations, yantras, mantras, mudras, meditation, mind training, identification & internalization of deities, mandalas, feasts, purification achievements, initiations, and more.

"Secrecy protects the tantric practitioner and his practice in several ways. It is said that the power and efficacy of the Vajrayana is dependent upon the devotion and respect of its practitioners. If one were to disclose to non-initiates one's practices and experiences, these would be met with misunderstanding and lack of appreciation, at the very least."

~ **Reginald A Ray,** *Secret of the Vajra World: The Tantric Buddhism of Tibet.*

Interestingly, the 6th Rite is very similar to Uddiyana Bandha, a Hatha yoga exercise which is commonly practised by men and women alike.

Here are Kelder's instructions on how to do the Sixth Rite:

- Stand erect and then let all the air out of the lungs, as one bends over and places his hands on his knees. Force out the last trace of air.

- Then, with empty lungs, stand erect, place hands on hips, and push down on them. This has a tendency to push up the shoulders.

- While doing this, pull in the abdomen just as far as possible, which raises the chest. Now hold this position as long as you can.

- Then when you are forced to take air into the empty lungs, let the air flow in through the nose.

- Exhale it through the mouth as you relax the arms and let them hang naturally at your sides.

- Then take several deep breaths through the mouth or nose and allow them to quickly escape through either the mouth or the nose.

- This constitutes one complete performance of Rite Number Six. About three are required to subdue the most powerful urge and to turn the powerful procreative or reproductive forces upward.

Uddiyana Bandha Instructions

In Hatha yoga it is recommended that you should only carry out uddiyana bandha on an empty stomach as the abdomen is contracted, up, and into the rib cage. It is performed only after an exhalation and never before an inhalation.

- ❑ Stand with your feet slightly apart and your knees bent.
- ❑ Round your torso forward with your hands resting on your knees.
- ❑ Inhale deeply, then exhale forcibly and quickly through your nose or mouth.
- ❑ Pull in (contract) your belly muscles to force as much air as possible out of your lungs.
- ❑ Relax your abdominals and expand your rib cage as though you were inhaling (but without the inhalation) – often called a "mock inhalation." This hollows the stomach, pulling it in and up towards the rib cage.
- ❑ Hold the bandha for about 5 – 15 seconds, then slowly release the grip and inhale normally.
- ❑ Between each repetition—around 3 to 10 depending on your capacity, take a few normal breaths.

LONG-LIVED LAMAS – PART THREE

15

After the tenth week Colonel Bradford no longer attended each weekly meeting. However, he still kept up his interest in the "Himalaya Club," and from time to time would speak on various subjects which would aid them in their work. Sometimes the members requested him to advise them on some particular subject. For instance, we discussed among ourselves one night the tremendously important part that food played in our lives. How the right food would make us more alive and vigorous while the wrong food would make us sluggish and dull. None of us knew much about the subject, however, so we requested the Colonel to advise us at our next meeting as to the Lamas' policy regarding food.

"In the Himalayan Lamasery where I was a neophyte," said the Colonel, in addressing us the following week, "there are no problems concerning the right foods, nor in getting sufficient food. Each of the Lamas does his share of the work in producing what is needed. Furthermore, all the work is done by the most primitive means. Even the soil is tiled by hand. Of course, the Lamas could use horses and plows if they so desired, but direct contact with the soil, handling it and working with it, seems to add something to man's existence. Personally, it made me feel very strongly that I was a part of the Universal. Not merely working with it or working for it but rather that the Universal and I were one.

"Now it is true that the Lamas are vegetarians, but not strictly so. They do use eggs, butter, and home-made cheese in quantities sufficient to serve certain functions of the brain, body, and nervous system. But aside from this they do not need meat, for all who are strong and virile, and who practice Rite Number Six have no need of meat, fish, or fowl.

"Most of those who join the ranks of the Lamas are men of the world who know little about proper food and diet. Yet they are only in the Grand Retreat in the Himalayas a very short while when they begin to show wonderful signs of physical improvement, due no doubt to the diet in the Lamasery.

"No Lama is choosy about his meals. He can't be because there is little to choose from. A Lama diet consists of good, wholesome food but as a rule it consists of but one article of food at a meal. That in itself is a secret of health. When one eats just one kind of food at a time there can be no clashing of foods in the stomach. Foods clash in the stomach because starches will not mix with proteins. For example, bread, which is starchy, when eaten with meats, eggs, or cheese, which are protein, sets up a reaction in the stomach which often causes not only immediate physical pain, but which contributes as well to a short life and a not particularly merry one.

"Many times in the Lamasery dining hall I have set down to the table along with the Lamas and eaten a meal consisting solely of bread. At other times I have had nothing but fresh vegetables and fresh fruits, while at still another meal I ate nothing but cooked vegetables and cooked fruits. At first I greatly missed the large variety of foods to which I had been accustomed; but after a short while I could eat and enjoy a meal consisting of nothing but dark bread or some one particular fruit. Sometimes it would be a feast of one vegetable.

"The point I wish to bring out to you gentlemen is not that you should resign yourselves to a diet of one kind of food to a meal but that you should keep starches, fruits, and vegetables separate from meats, fish, and fowl at your meals.

"It is permissible to make a meal of just meat. In fact, you could have several kinds of meats to a meal. You can have butter, eggs, and cheese with the meat meal, and dark bread, and, if you wish, coffee, or tea, but you must not end up with anything sweet or starchy. No pies or cakes or puddings.

"Then again, your meal can be strictly starches. Then you can indulge in all the sweet fruits, all the bread, butter, pies, cakes, puddings, and fresh or cooked vegetables you like without feeling any ill effects. But keep these meals separate.

"Butter seems to be a neutral. It can be used with either a starchy meal or with a meat meal. Milk, however, agrees better with starch meals.

"The proper use of eggs was another interesting and beneficial thing that came to my attention while dwelling in the Lamasery. The Lamas would not eat whole eggs unless they were engaged in hard manual labor; then they might eat one, medium-boiled. However, they did indulge to a very great extent in raw egg yolks, discarding the white part. Before I learned better it seemed a waste of perfectly good food to toss the cooked whites of the egg back to the chickens, but now I know that no one should eat the whites of eggs unless he is doing hard manual labor; the egg whites are used only by the muscles.

"Although I had always been aware of the fact that egg yolks were particularly good for one, it wasn't until after I arrived at the Lamasery and had an opportunity to talk with an old Austrian chemist that I learned their true value. Then I was amazed to find out that just common hen eggs contain at least half of the sixteen elements required by the brain, blood, nerves, and tissues. It is true that these elements are only needed in small quantities, but they must be included in the diet if one is to be exceptionally robust and healthy, both mentally and physically.

"There is one thing more of great importance that I learned from the Lamas. They taught me to eat, not slowly for its own sake, but so that I might masticate my food more thoroughly. Their bread is tough and it takes good chewing to reduce it to a liquid before swallowing it, but this I learned to do.

"Everything one eats should be 'digested,' so to speak, in the mouth before allowing it to enter the stomach. Starches, particularly, must be digested in the mouth. Unless they first are thoroughly mixed with saliva they literally are dynamite when they get to the stomach.

"While one can do with little mastication of protein foods, such as meat, fish, and fowl, it is a sensible thing to chew them well anyhow. More nourishment can be obtained from food when it is thoroughly masticated. This necessitates less food, and often the amount can be reduced by one-half.

"Many things which I had casually taken for granted before entering the Lamasery seemed shocking when I left it two years later. One of the first things I noted upon arriving in one of the larger cities in India was the prodigious amount of food consumed by everyone who could afford to do so. I have seen one man eat a quantity of food at a meal sufficient to feed four hard-working Lamas and keep them thriving.

"Variety was another thing which appalled me. Having been in the habit of eating but one or two foods at a meal, it amazed me to count 23 varieties of food one evening on my host's table. No wonder that the English and the Americans have such miserable stomachs and such damnably poor health.

They seem to know nothing whatsoever about the kind of food they should eat for health and strength.

"Just the other evening I had dinner with a very learned man. He was an educator and quite an intellectual. He calmly stated, while we waited to be served, that in a few short years the human race could become really worthwhile providing his ideas were thoroughly carried out.

"This man was an excellent dictator type, and I was quite impressed by his knowledge, his original ideas, and his ability to express himself. But when I saw this man's selection of food at the dinner table, my opinion of him changed. It was the most atrocious combination of unnutritive TNT I ever saw. I thought, if I could only give him some simple ideas about food he could become a really worthwhile force for good in the world in a short time.

"The right food, the right combinations of foods, the right amount of food, and the right method of eating food combines to do great things for one. It will enable one to put on weight if he is underweight, and to reduce if he is overweight. Keep in mind these five things:

"Never eat starch and meat at the same meal; although if you are strong and healthy it need not cause you too much concern now.

If coffee bothers you, drink it black, using no milk or cream. If it bothers you then, discontinue its use.

Chew your food to a liquid and cut down on the amount as much as possible.

By all means and before all else eat raw egg yolks once a day, every day. Take them at meal times but not with after.

Reduce the varieties of food to a minimum. If one is really hungry before he starts eating, the tendency to desire many different foods is lost in hunger."

"It is a very simple matter," continued Colonel Bradford, "to live simply in this highly complex world. Let the world be complex but let your diet, and all matters pertaining to your mental and physical wellbeing be simple. One can do this and still lead a very active life in the modern world. Not all Lamas in India live constantly in Lamaseries. Many of them are found in the cities where they are engaged in professions, or are at the head of great business institutions. These men, like their brother Lamas in secluded Lamaseries, live to amazing ages – amazing to the Western World, but quite a commonplace thing in the East. Just how old these Lamas are I do not know from first-hand experience, but I have been reliably informed that some of them remain in the flesh in a hale and hearty condition five to ten times longer than do most people of the Western World."

VOICES, VORTEXES, AND VITALITY – PART FOUR

16

Colonel Bradford was speaking before the "Himalaya Club" for the last time before leaving on a tour of the United States and a visit to his native England. He had selected for his subject the things that help youthify a man, regardless of whether or not he practices Rite Number Six. As the Colonel spoke he seemed to be keener, more alert and vigorous and virile than ever before. Upon his return from the Lamasery he had struck me as the acme of perfection; yet since then he had kept right on improving, and even now was making new gains constantly.

"There are several things I want to talk about tonight;" began the Colonel, "which I am sure will interest you. The first of them is the human voice. Do you realize that when one has made a study of men's voices he can tell instantly how much masculine vitality a man possesses just by hearing him speak? You have all heard the shrill, piping voice of an old man. Well, when a man's voice begins to take on that high pitch he is in a very deplorable condition. Let me explain.

"The Vortex at the base of the neck has power over the vocal cords. This Vortex and the one in the sex center are connected. Of course, all the Vortexes have a common connection, but these two are geared together, as it were. What affects one affects the other, so that when a man's voice is high his manly vitality is low. (I am not speaking of Tenor voices.)

"Now all that is necessary to speed up these two Vortexes, along with the others, is to practice the Five Rites. However, one does not have to wait until these Vortexes are increased in speed by the use of the Five Rites, but can raise their speed of vibration with a special method that works very well. This particular practice is easy. It consists of simply putting forth an effort to keep the voice masculine; not allowing it to become high, shrill, or piping. Listen to men with good low voices and become conscious of how a real man's voice sounds. Then whenever you talk, keep the voice down to the masculine vibration.

"Real old men will find this to be quite a little task; but it brings results. The first thing you know the lowered voice will speed up the Vortex in the base of the throat. That will speed up the Vortex in the sex center, which will improve the man in masculine energy, and this again will cause the Vortex in the throat to speed up. The adolescent boy whose voice is changing is experiencing the same thing. The Two Vortexes are speeding up. In this case it is usually caused by the Vortex in the procreative center being speeded up by nature. But anything that will speed up the Vortex in the throat will cause its companion Vortex immediately below to increase speed.

"There are a number of young men who are robust and virile now who will not remain that way long. This is due to the fact that their particular voice, for several reasons I haven't the time to explain now, never came down to the masculine pitch. But these young men, as well as the old ones, can definitely get results of a very wonderful nature by consciously lowering their voices. In the young men it will mean prolonged virility; in the older men, renewed virility.

"Some time ago I came across a quite splendid voice exercise. Like all other potent things it is very simple. Whenever you are by yourself or where there is sufficient noise to drown your voice so that you will not annoy others, practice saying in low tones, partly through the nose:

"Me - me - me - me - e - e - e - e - e - e - e - e - e."

"Repeat it time and again. When you get it down quite low, try it in a small room, like the bath room. You can often make the room hum with your voice. Then try to get the same effect in a larger room. Of course, listening to this vibration of your voice is not entirely necessary; but often the vibration will cause the other Vortexes in the body to speed up, especially the one in the sex center and the two in the head.

"The 'Me - me - e - e - e -' exercise is a good one, but you can use to good advantage other vowels, also. 'Mo mo - o- o - o - o' as well as 'Ma - ma- ma - a - a - a', and 'Mu - mu- mu- u- u- u- u' are good. Like the e's on 'me', and the o's in 'Mo', the a's in 'Ma' and the u's in 'Mu' are drawn out very long as a single sound and not as so many short ones. Each of the vowel sounds should be started with 'M', and the 'M' should be repeated with the vowel three or four times, then draw out the vowel into a long one. Always start with the 'Me - me - me - e - e - e - e' exercise and end with the 'Mu - mu - mu - u - u - u - u' exercise. Start with the first and repeat it twenty-five times, then go on to the others – each twenty-five times. Some students get the best results from the use of the 'Me me - me - e - e - e' practice only.

"In old women, the voice also becomes shrill and should be toned down. Of course, a woman's voice naturally is higher than a man's. If she should get it down as low as a man's, it would not be beneficial at all to her. It would speed up the Two Vortexes – the one in the throat and its companion, so as to cause her to act, look, think, and talk mannishly. By the same token, a mannish woman could wonderfully improve herself by raising her voice to the level of a normal woman's.

"I have known of men with high voices who partook of so much alcoholic beverages that they developed 'whiskey' voices – low and growling. To their amazement they began to become virile again. Usually they attributed their good fortune to intemperance or to a certain brand of whiskey, but neither intemperance nor whiskey did anything for them directly.

"What happened was that the vocal cords were irritated and therefore inflamed and swollen. This lowered the voice and raised the speed of the Vortex in the throat, which in turn, raised the vibrations of the Vortex in the masculine center below, and brought about the renewed masculine vitality.

"Now," said the Colonel, after pausing a moment, "I want to speak on one more subject, which could be entitled 'Putting off the old man.' Lowering the voice and speeding up the Vortexes certainly has a lot to do in eliminating the 'old man' within us, but there are other things which help to make us much younger even though they do not directly affect the Vortexes. If it were possible suddenly to take a man out of a decrepit old body and place him in a brand-new youthful one about 25 years of age, I am confident that the old man he had allowed himself to become would cause him to remain old in most of his ways. It is true that he would perk up a bit around the ladies; outside of that I think he would remain old.

"Getting old, of course, is brought about first by a lack or a complete absence of manly virility. But that is not the only cause. The world is full of old men around 60 who get a certain dubious pleasure out of acting old. This is all wrong. Regardless of whether a man has full vitality at the present time or not, he should do everything possible to eliminate the 'old man' that has crept within him. He must be dislodged and rooted out. Therefore, gentlemen, from now on get rid of the 'old man' within you. How to do it? It is very simple. Don't do the things old people do. With your new and ever-increasing vitality this should be easy.

"The first thing to do is to straighten up. Stand like a man should. When you first started this class, some of you were so bent over that you looked like question marks; but as vigor returned and spirits became better you began to straighten up. That was fine; but don't stop now. Straighten right on up, start throwing your chest out, pull the stomach and the chin in, and right away you have eliminated 20 years from your appearance and 40 years from your mind. Likewise, eliminate the 'old man' mannerisms. When you walk, know first where you are going; then start out and go there. Don't dog-trot or run, and don't shuffle along, but pick up your feet and stride. Keep one eye on where you are going and the other one on everything you pass.

"At the Himalayan Lamasery there was a man, a European, whom you would have sworn was not over 35 years of age, and who acted like a man of 25 in every respect. This man was over a hundred, and if I told you how much over a hundred you would not believe me.

"Now about your weight. If you are underweight, you can throw off the years by increasing your weight. If you are overweight, which is a splendid sign of old age and senility, you can throw off more years by reducing the weight to normal. Get rid of the enlarged abdomens, too, and you will look 10 years younger immediately.

"Here is something else which should interest all of you. Only two years ago I was as bald as the baldest man here. When vitality started coming back, one of the Lamas told me to massage my scalp good with a piece of butter twice a week. The butter up there was fresh, not a bit of salt in it. I took his advice and massaged my scalp with butter until it soon loosened up.

I did this about one hour after a meal. The food elements in the blood were brought to the scalp by the circulation of the blood. The scalp was so thoroughly massaged that the blood vessels were dilated; the hair roots picked up the necessary nutrition, and the hair grew, as you can plainly see.

"Even though you may not care to become mystics at this time, you can throw many years off your mind, your attitude, and feelings. So start at once. Any effort you put forth will be rewarded, I can assure you. I have given you nothing but simple Rites and practices because the simple things will bring you health, youth, virility, and success when nothing else will.

"It has been a most thrilling thing to see you men change and improve from day to day," concluded the Colonel, "but now you know all there is need for you to know for the present. When you are ready for more information, the teacher will appear. There are others who need this information much more than you gentlemen did and I must be on my way to them."

Of course, we were sorry to see our friend the Colonel depart. But we were glad and thankful for the priceless information he had given us. The thought that the Colonel was soon to help other men like ourselves find "The Fountain of Youth," "The Philosopher's Stone," "The Elixir of Life," thrilled us. Truly, I thought to myself, THE EYE OF REVELATION is upon the world.

Note: *In 1946, Peter Kelder republished 'The Eye of Revelation' with amendments, and a whole new Chapter containing information on 'Mantram-Mind Magic' and 'The Magic Quality of AUM.'*

1946 EDITION – THE EYE OF REVELATION

by Peter Kelder

"THE EYE OF REVELATION" is an Education and Inspiration Course of Study, and of Practice.

"THE EYE OF REVELATION" is intended for men and women everywhere throughout the Western World, and this regardless of nationality.

'THE EYE OF REVELATION" is intended for the personal use of the purchaser of this Course only. It may not be loaned or given to any other person, except members of one's own, immediate family.

'THE EYE OF REVELATION' is intended only for those who are mentally and physically capable of performing the various exercises or rites contained in this book or monograph. The Author and Publishers are therefore, in no way responsible for the misuse of any of the information which is contained herein.

$2.00 the Copy Postpaid

THE MID-DAY PRESS
1045 Midway Place
Los Angeles 15,
California

17

MANTRAM-MIND MAGIC – PART FIVE

Now and then the "Himalaya Club" would receive a short but interesting communication from Colonel Bradford. He did not stay long in any one place, and so the "Club" knew that he was traveling about and lecturing before other groups throughout the English-speaking world.

One day the "Himalaya Club" received quite a long letter from the Colonel. It contained additional information, and was intended for all of the members. Probably only the more advanced members would be sufficiently interested in it to put it to use.

The title of the subject was: "Mantram-Mind Magic". The word Mantram, as far as the meaning was concerned, was entirely new to the group, although some of the members vaguely remembered seeing it somewhere in print.

Colonel Bradford's letter explained:

"A Mantram is a 'vocalized instrument of thought'. There is a slight difference between Mantram and Mantra. Usually, Mantram means vocalized thought, while Mantra is an inaudible thought.

"Time and again, each of you has had some word or group of words 'run through your mind'. Sometimes it would be only one word, at other times it would be two words, or a short group of words. Often it would be the name of something, or probably some one's name. When something of such a nature keeps running through your mind it is a Mantra — an inaudible instrument of thought. Just how it got started we haven't the space to go into here, and furthermore it is not important to know the cause at this time.

"The important thing is to take advantage of this subconscious activity, and this can easily be done when you know how. This is how you proceed: The moment you become aware of something running through your mind in the form of definite words (not a tune), vocalize it. Let us say that the thought was 'peace in our time'. Now each time the thought — 'peace in our time' — passes through your mind, vocally repeat the thought and add another one to it like this. 'Peace in our time', means peace, power and plenty for me right now. In this way you take a deep-seated sub-conscious activity and attach to it something of meaning and consequence, and after a while when the subconscious ceases to project its activity into your conscious mind, although it will continue to repeat the thought within itself (this has been proven through the use of hypnotism) it will repeat along with its own your added thought, and instead of repeating over and over again, 'peace in our time', it will repeat 'Peace in our time means peace, power and plenty for me right now'.

"Before too long a time by proceeding in this manner your sub-conscious realm of mind will be so 'galvanized' with the meaning of the new thought that you attached to the sub-conscious thought that the sub-conscious mind will begin to put the thought into practice in your conscious life, and the result will be a quieting of the things that disturb you through the word 'peace', and this regardless of what the disturbing elements might consist.

"Don't try to figure out how the sub-conscious is going to overcome certain obstacles in your life and affairs to bring about peace in your life. The sub-conscious in its way is far more clever than is our conscious realm of mind. The conscious mind is always coming up against stone walls, just can't go any further in that direction, and soon hasn't the energy to attempt to go in any other direction, but not so with the subconscious mind. The sub-conscious is not a reasoning mind and so if it is headed-off in one direction it is not discouraged, doesn't give up, because it knows (feels) that there are ten thousand other directions that it can turn, and at least half of that number will permit it to bring about the desired results in YOUR Life and affairs.

"We said that a Mantram was a vocalized instrument of thought. Use a Mantram whenever you can, because the vocalization of the thought causes you to hear it, and this means an additional impression upon the sub-conscious. The idea is to send just as powerful a suggestion into the sub-conscious realm of mind as possible.

"On the other hand, if we are in close contact with other people, as we are when riding along in a train with fellow passengers sitting all about us and even another in the same seat with us, we can't very well speak out and say 'Peace in our time means peace, power and plenty for me right now'. In such a case I would suggest that we use a Mantra, and quietly think to ourself 'Peace in our time means peace, power and plenty for me right now'. True, it will not be quite as effective, but we still will get splendid results.

"Even after the sub-conscious has ceased projecting such a thought into our conscious mind it is a very fine idea to continue the work for some time to come, and every two or three minutes repeat the suggestion along with the subconscious thought of 'Peace in our time'. The 'peace in our time' of the sub-conscious is the OPEN DOOR to the subconscious, and this 'door' remains open for a considerable time after the thought rises high enough to contact our conscious mind.

"Always make your additions to your sub-conscious thought positive, short, and to the point. We explained about the word 'peace', how it brings about desirable results to you. Well, the word 'power', when taken deep into the sub-consciousness will one day bring about health, strength and vitality in our physical bodies, and not only that, we will find that we are actually becoming much more self-controlled, and dominant mentally.

"The word 'plenty' in our suggestion of course means abundance. You not only want peace, but you want an abundance of peace. You are not satisfied with just a little power in body and mind, you want an abundance of it.

"'Right now' at the end of your affirmation gives the subconscious mind some ideas as to when you want all of this to materialize — N-O-W. You desire that the sub-conscious mind start bringing about the desired changes at once. Not a week, or a month, or a year from now, but get busy and cause them to come into manifestation in your life and affairs now.

"The sub-conscious thought will be anything of a million different thoughts or half-thoughts. Sometimes they are the names or [of?] people; other times, the names of plays you have seen either recently or some time ago; or perhaps they will be the names of stories or books. It doesn't matter what the thought is that persists in running through your mind, just add another one to it and everytime [sic] the thought comes to mind repeat the thought that comes to mind, and then attach your thought — your affirmation -to it.

"A long time ago you probably read the book 'Jane Eyre", or saw the film version of it. Now, for no apparent reason (although there is a good sub-conscious one) the thought 'Jane Eyre' runs through your mind time and time again. Well, just the moment you become aware of it just repeat it and add a thought to it: 'Jane Eyre' means peace, power and plenty to me right now.

"It is wise to place the word means between the sub-conscious thought and your added thought. This informs the subconsciousness in a very short and definite way YOUR MEANING of 'Jane Eyre'. It is necessary to be very definite with the subconscious mind, for in certain respects it is quite child-like, and it must have definite thoughts if you expect it to do its best work.

"No matter what words or phrases run through your mind — 'peace in our time', 'Jane Eyre', 'Wee Willie Winkle', etc., etc., just add YOUR MEANING to them, and as the subconscious activity withdraws itself into the sub-conscious the thoughts, regardless of what they are, will have YOUR THOUGHT attached to them, and it is your thought that will do the miracles in your subconscious world for you. [sic] Not only in your sub-conscious world but a little later on in your CONSCIOUS or OUTER WORLD.

"By all means make up your own affirmations or autosuggestions to suit yourself. While 'peace, power and plenty right now' is good, there is probably something else that you need more than these three. Whatever it is, make it into an affirmation and hook it onto your sub-conscious Mantra to be drawn deep into your sub-conscious world, and put to work.

"Some folks have a sub-conscious mind that is very close to the surface of the conscious mind, and the result is, never a week passes but what they have some subconscious thought running through their conscious mind time and again. If you are one of these people, then about once a week you'll be able to give your sub-conscious realm of mind a very excellent treatment of suggestions or affirmations.

"There are other folks whose sub-conscious is not 'located' so near to the conscious mind and, they seldom if ever have a thought run through their minds hour upon hour or even for a few minutes. These folks, however, can induce the sub-conscious to come to the surface with a thought to which an affirmation can be added.

"Just a catchy little phrase like 'Wee Willie Winkle', if thought to one's self for a short period of time will in most instances cause the sub-conscious to open the door between itself and the conscious mind, and every few seconds repeat 'Wee Willie Winkle', and after a little of this (do not begin too soon) start adding whatever you desire 'Wee Willie Winkle' to mean.

"The sub-conscious realm of mind is a very wonderful 'creation' and it is not half as hard to get it to work with you as to get you to work with it. In fact, the sub-conscious takes great delight in working with you in accomplishing anything that you desire. Desire is a very strong force, and when you use desire to induce the sub-conscious to bring about certain desirable results in your life, it will actually be thrilled to work with you, to actually go out and get the things that you want, to cause the desires of your heart to be realized or materialized.

"This is something that each of you should know: The sub-conscious realm of mind cannot feel pain or sorrow or grief. None of these feelings or emotions are unpleasant to it, would be a better way of stating the matter. Your pain is a thrilling sensation to the sub-conscious. Your joy, enthusiasm, zeal and fervor, also are thrilling sensations to your sub-conscious mind, but as misery is much easier for each one of us to experience than is joy, quite naturally the only real pleasure the sub-conscious gets, and it is a joy-loving 'creature', is from our pain, sorrow and misery, and quite naturally it brings about these unpleasant things in our lives 'thinking' that we get as much pleasure from them as does 'it' — the sub-conscious mind.

"Once we convince the sub-consciousness that we get our big thrills out of the joyous things of life, the subconscious will flood our lives with the thrilling things instead of the miserable things of life.

THE MAGIC
QUALITY OF AUM

18

" To a person who doesn't know English, an affirmation such as 'peace, power and plenty right now' wouldn't mean a thing to his sub-conscious mind, unless it was translated into his own language, and he could use words that he was highly familiar with which meant 'peace, power and plenty right now'.

"I mention this because certain teachers from the East have given out certain affirmations which are very fine to people who know the language of the East. But these affirmations are absolutely worthless to English-speaking people because they do not know the meaning of the words or phrases. Even if they have been told the meaning, the words are still just so much jargon to the sub-conscious, and the result is, no good is accomplished. The subconscious is a wonderful thing, but it cannot possibly use thoughts that are enshrouded in foreign words unless these words are <u>completely familiar to you</u>.

"There is one exception, however — a word that comes from the East which has a magical effect upon the subconscious as well as upon the brain and nervous system. This word is 'aum'. The value of the word is not in its meaning but in its vibration. Thus, anyone using it for vibratory purposes, regardless of which particular language of earth [sic] he speaks, will receive a special benefit from it; that is, of course, if he is ready for a high and powerful vibration. Nothing is good or beneficial if its vibration is so great that it is wholly out of harmony with a lesser vibration.

"This particular word — aum — when vibrated correctly, has a very powerful stimulating effect upon the pineal gland, but, the pineal gland should not be stimulated into great action if the life a person is leading is not on a high plane. A person should be sufficiently high in his vibrations through right living that he is beyond the use of habit-forming drugs, which include alcohol and nicotine in any and all forms.

"One's diet should be minus, to a considerable extent (but not entirely), fats of all kinds but especially lard. Meat is permissible in sensible and limited quantities, but <u>pork in any form should be dispensed with</u>. A small amount of butter is permissible. White sugar as well as all foods containing large quantities of white sugar should be used sparingly. Honey and natural sweets can be used instead and even they should not be over-indulged in. They are too sugar [sic], and sugar is a first-cousin to alcohol, and alcohol is completely OUT when one is attempting to travel the path of the thrilling higher vibrations.

"Starches, too, are detrimental unless they are well masticated — practically digested in the mouth — then they are no longer harmful if taken in sensible quantities.

"The average, normal man consumes about two quarts of water each twenty-four hours. A woman weighing less naturally consumes less liquid. The consumption of water should be increased considerably. A man should increase the intake of water from two quarts per day to three, and a woman should increase her consumption of liquid from one quart per day to one and a half. Even a little more for both men and women would be still better. However, the increased amount of water should not be made all at once, but over a period of at least two months, and of course no change at all in the amount of liquid if a person is ailing physically, without permission from their physician.

"The increased use of water should take place first, and for at least a month, then one can use the Aum-Vibration Rite for good results.

"The 'au' in AUM is pronounced 'ah'. It is pronounced through the mouth and is drawn out for about <u>five seconds</u>, then the mouth is closed (not suddenly) and the 'm' is hummed out through the nose (either nostril) for <u>ten seconds</u>.

"After a breath or two, then do the 'au-m-m-m-m-m' again. Three or four times in succession is quite sufficient. Do not overdo a good thing. Stop the moment you begin to feel dizzy. After an hour or so perform the 'aum's' again several times. At first never more than ten times even though no sign of any dizziness has become manifest. Too much pineal stimulation for a beginner is not a positive procedure.

"The best position to take for this Rite is to sit in an easy chair and completely relax. Don't slouch down so that your head will thrust forward and cramp your vocal cords. It is necessary to get a good clear tone both through the mouth and through the nose, and if you are in a cramped position you cannot do this.

"One can even lie flat on the back on a comfortable bed or divan and perform this Rite to splendid advantage. The pillow should be removed so that one can get the head far enough back in order that the vocal cords will not be cramped.

"Don't fill the lungs bursting full of air, but amply sufficient to do the Aum-Vibration for fifteen seconds (five seconds through the mouth — ten seconds through the nose) without being completely out of breath at the end of the 15 seconds.

"Like in the Mantra and Mantram Rites, you can use an affirmation in this Mantram-Aum Rite to splendid advantage.

"You will remember that in the Mantra Rite you repeat your affirmation mentally. In the Mantram Rite you repeat the affirmation vocally. This one is a combination of both of the other Rites. While you are vocalizing 'ah' in aum for five seconds you <u>hold the mind quiet</u>, then while you are intoning the 'm' through the nose for ten seconds <u>you repeat your affirmation mentally several times</u>.

"It is best not to use this Rite and the previous one at the same time. Use this one when the mind is free from any sub-conscious thoughts running through it.

"Also: It is best to prepare your affirmation before you begin to practice the Aum Rite, so you will know exactly what to suggest. Be sure that it contains exactly that which you wish to become or that which you desire. Be absolutely certain that the affirmation does not contain any negative thoughts or words, in this way you will not build into your sub-consciousness anything of a detrimental character.

"Always remember that while you are humming the 'm' in <u>aum</u> through the nose (mouth closed) you, with your mental affirmation, are making a powerful impression on your sub-conscious mind, so powerful in fact that your words and your thoughts are being permanently etched upon it, and for this reason you most certainly do not want anything negative in your affirmation. If you do, eventually it will come to the surface mind, and you will have lost all the good which you could otherwise have accomplished.

"This Rite is intended for older people only. It most certainly is not to be used by persons under twenty-one years of age. It is intended for mature men and women. Especially those who have not found life a bed of roses. It is for those who wish to 'reclaim the years that the locusts have eaten'.

"The Illuminati — the Wise Men of old — have all used this unusual form of Mantra or Mantram for raising the vibration of not only their minds and brains, but their physical bodies as well. The Rite has a most beneficial effect on all of the old-age-producing causes in the physical body — by eliminating them, of course. Quite naturally if we refuse to eliminate any of the known old-age producers in mind and body we can not expect to get thrilling results from this particular Rite. But as causes for old age and senility are eliminated we can rest assured that the vibrations of our minds and bodies will be increased, and then we shall go forward to youth of mind and youth of body, and there is nothing more thrilling than a <u>mature</u> young mind in a renewed body.

"One reason why older people make so much better progress, once they start to increase their vibrations than do men and women one-half or even one-third of their age, is due to the fact that they have finally learned that the materialistic world is just a make-shift, make-believe existence, and any joys found in it are as fleeting as dry leaves in a windstorm. They know that the Great Thrills of Life are not found in the outer world, but in the Inner World — in their INNER WORLD. And, once they begin to experience the thrill of the higher vibrations working in their minds and bodies, nothing could ever induce them to go back into the senseless lives they lived before they ever heard of an Inner World.

"The Eye of Revelation is upon you. Great days are ahead for all of us, and this regardless of present conditions or circumstances. Begin anew right where you are, and even though most of you have made gratifying accomplishments, these are as nothing in comparison to the thrilling things that are just a short distance ahead of you."

Aum, also known as "OM," is believed to be the first sound heard from the creator at the beginning of the universe. It is said that this primordial sound is the original sound that contains all other sounds, all words, all languages, and all mantras.

A mantra assists your mind to focus when it is scattered. When you chant a mantra, it produces a powerful vibration that can eventually still all other vibrations, although it takes a lot of practice to achieve this. The purpose of a mantra is to produce a state by which you are able to vibrate at the same rate as the energy and spiritual state produced by and contained within the mantra.

Om is commonly chanted at the beginning and end of a yoga class to attune yourself to the universal consciousness – you can do the same with the Rites. It allows us to experience our connection or reflection as part of the whole. It can be chanted at any other suitable time, at a length to be determined by the individual chanter, which meets his or her level of total comfort, provided it does not strain the lungs. According to Hindu scriptures, the highest experience in life is to hear the sound of OM in deep silence. The repetition of OM is said to generate the mystical power that can lead your mind into deep meditation and finally into the state of higher consciousness known as Samadhi (bliss).

- *To chant AUM, you begin with a deep breath.*
- *Then, in an effortless single out-breath, the sound A (as in awe) originates in the navel, then rises to the throat with the U (as in OO), opens the fontanelle at the top of the head, and ends with MMMM, which rolls over the tongue with your front teeth lightly touching at the final point.*
- *At the beginning of the chant, there is an expansion outwards, which ends with a contraction inwards at the conclusion of the M sound.*
- *Then repeat again and again as desired.*

CHOOSING THE RIGHT METHOD FOR YOU

F it or not, I recommend you follow Colonel Bradford's advice by beginning with three repetitions (of each Rite) per day in your first week. Then, every week, add two more repetitions of each Rite like this –

Week Two – 5 reps per day of Rites 1-5

Week Three – 7 reps per day of Rites 1-5

Week Four – 9 reps per day of Rites 1-5

Week Five – 11 reps per day and so on

Following the monks' instructions, you will reach the required 21 repetitions in ten weeks. This may seem like a long time to get to 21, but I can assure you the arrival at your destination will be all the richer for having undergone the journey to get there.

Your body needs time to adjust to changes to your balance system and energy system. Building up repetitions too quickly can create a detox effect as well as a degree of dizziness or nausea. These side effects can be improved or avoided altogether by gradually increasing your repetitions.

Remember this isn't just physical exercise – the true purpose of the Rites as described by Kelder is:

"The body has seven centers, which, in English, could be called Vortexes. These are kind of magnetic centers. They revolve at great speed in the healthy body, but when slowed down – well that is just another name for old age, ill-health, and senility. These spinning centers of activity extend beyond the flesh in the healthy individual, but in the old, weak, senile person they hardly reach the surface, except in the knees. The quickest way to regain health, youth, and vitality is to start these magnetic centers spinning again. There are but five practices that will do this. Any one of them will be helpful, but all five are required to get glowing results. These five exercises are really not exercises at all, in the physical culture sense. The Lamas think of them as 'Rites' and so instead of calling them exercises or practices, we too, shall call them 'Rites'."

~ **Peter Kelder,** *The Eye of Revelation.*

LEARNING THE RITES

Throughout these pages, I have shared some of my knowledge about teaching The Five Tibetan Rites for the last twenty-three years. However, this book was never intended to be a complete instructional manual - its purpose was to share the unadulterated words of Peter Kelder and share some useful tips.

Obviously, there is a lot more I can share with you, but for now, here is a brief overview of what I have learned in case you want to know more.

I call the way I teach the Rites "T5T" because it is a lot quicker than saying "The Five Tibetan Rites." It also provides a means for people to identify this method of learning the Rites, which has been tried and tested by so many thousands of students.

For many people, the descriptions inside this book are sufficient to learn the Rites - generally, those of you who are younger, fitter, have good body-mind awareness and have not suffered from a back or neck injury in the past.

The Five Tibetan Rites are repetitive movements, and there are some key points to be aware of to avoid strain or injury – particularly if you want to establish a long-term practice. Rest assured, if you were to learn the Rites by the T5T method, you would experience exactly the same benefits as everyone else. However, you would also have additional benefits – significant improvements to core strength and breathing capacity.

T5T is for those who want more in-depth instructions than this book's limited ones. It is for anyone who needs to learn how to move their body safely while carrying out repetitive movements daily – or for anyone needing modifications or adaptations due to muscle weakness or injury. Most of all, T5T is for those who want to protect and strengthen their body's vulnerable areas, lower backs, and necks – not just when doing the Rites, but during their everyday life too.

One of the principal things we have learned from fine-tuning solutions to solve students' common problems is the importance of developing strong core muscles to protect the spine. It is also the key to a successful long-term practice and a short-term pleasurable learning experience.

Consider this: *When you have built up to 21 repetitions of each movement (five postures performed 21 times each), you will be doing 105 repetitions per day. Over a year (365 days), that is 38,325 repetitions. As you can imagine, it is vital to have correct alignment and technique*

- *Core muscles are the deepest muscles closest to the spine, and when correctly activated, they wrap around and protect the spine like a natural weight belt or girdle.*

  (a) *The first step is learning to correctly identify and activate your core muscles. It is easy to use the stronger, more external muscles of the abdomen instead, leaving the inner muscles underdeveloped (like a soft-centered chocolate.)*

  (b) *To achieve core strength, we follow the 10-week build-up recommendations of the monks mentioned earlier but include a variation in how we do the 2nd Rite (the Leg Raise) every week.*

  (c) *Just like lifting weights at the gym: You begin with low loads (in our case, the natural weight of the legs) and gradually increase the load and repetitions by shifting from single-leg to double-leg movements or from bent legs to straight legs.*

- *We incorporate **natural full breathing** when practicing the Rites (and between each Rite) due to the great benefits optimal breathing provides to vitality and health.*

- *For people who cannot do the Rites exactly as described, we provide **modifications** that do not reduce the benefits of the Rites in any way.*

"**T5T** is an incredible and powerful program. It turns back the clock. It increases your energy, mental clarity, and focus. It reduces stress and improves strength and flexibility. It is capable of restoring your passion and zest for life if you let it. I highly recommend it for anyone willing to improve their life."

~ John Gray ~
Author of *Men are from Mars, Women are from Venus*

THINGS TO BE CONSIDERED BEFORE LEARNING THE RITES

Are you currently doing very little exercise?	YES/NO
Have you ever practiced yoga before?	YES/NO
Have you suffered from back pain or neck pain in the past?	YES/NO
Have you seen any therapist for back or neck pain in the past?	YES/NO
Is one side of your body (or one limb) noticeably stronger than the other?	YES/NO
Have you noticed any muscular weakness in any part of your body?	YES/NO
Have you noticed any stiffness in any part of your body?	YES/NO
Do you find it an effort to maintain an upright stance when sitting or standing? Do you slouch?	YES/NO
Do you hold tension in your shoulders and upper back?	YES/NO
Weak or inflexible wrists. Do you find it a bit of a struggle to unscrew jars/bottles etc.?	YES/NO
Do you find it difficult to turn your neck around sufficiently when reversing your car?	YES/NO
Are you overweight?	YES/NO
Are you largely sedentary? You spend most of your time sitting in front of a desk or relaxing at home?	YES/NO
Are you at a point where you think you had better 'do' something now, before it is too late?	YES/NO

MORE YES ANSWERS THAN NO?

Fit or Relatively Fit?

Would you describe your level of fitness as being good across all four levels below?

Muscle tone ☐
Flexibility & range of motion ☐
Body awareness ☐
Energy & stamina ☐

Is core stability part of your workout? YES/NO

Are you able to identify and isolate each core muscle; the pelvic floor, transversus abdominis & multifidus muscles. YES/NO

Do you know when or if you incorrectly use your obliques to stabilise rather than your core muscles? YES/NO

Do you know how to establish and maintain neutral spine and neutral pelvis, whilst keeping your head and neck in line with your spine? YES/NO

How good is your breathing? If you already practice pranayama, are you also aware of what natural, full breathing should feel like. Consider this:

a. *Are all your breathing spaces able to open when breathing fully? Wide to the side, the back, the front, the ribs?*
b. *Do you have tension/tightness in your breathing?*
c. *How are your stress levels? Do you find yourself breathing rapidly into the upper chest, holding your breath, yawning or sighing?*
d. *Anders Ollson of Conscious Breathing is an expert at improving our breathing habits - you can try his free online breathing tests to check out how well you breathe.*
YES/NO

Having completed this questionnaire, you should have a better idea of which method of learning the 5 Tibetan Rites is best for you. Many people begin practicing by following the instructions in this book, but if you want more detailed explanations and alternatives, you might prefer to learn the T5T version.

If you have previously suffered back, neck, shoulder, hip, or wrist pain, consider learning the T5T method, which has adaptations and modifications you can use. T5T also incorporates core stability to strengthen the muscles that support and protect the spine. See also the chapter on "Health Considerations."

Regardless of which method you use, you will find answers to frequently asked questions, resources, information, and interesting articles on my T5T website.

If you would like to join a group of fellow practitioners on Facebook, or connect with the author – see details at the back of the book.

AFTERWORD

The Tibetan way of life today is unrecognizable from the one 'Colonel Bradford' described in 1939. Just ten years later, in 1949, Mao Zedong proclaimed the founding of the People's Republic of China and threatened to 'liberate' Tibet. In 1951 Tibetan leaders were forced to sign a treaty agreeing to the establishment of Chinese civil and military headquarters in Lhasa, but mounting resentment against Chinese rule led to armed resistance, leading to a full-scale uprising in Lhasa in 1959. During the suppression of the revolt, where thousands are said to have died, the Dalai Lama, most of his ministers, and around 80,000 other Tibetans fled to Dharamsala in India, where they have remained ever since.

According to the Tibetan Government in Exile, an estimated 1.2 million Tibetans have died as a direct result of Chinese occupation, and over 6,000 monasteries, temples and countless sacred texts and religious artifacts have been destroyed.

Today, China continues to falsely state that Tibet has always been part of the motherland and claims that they have brought progress to Tibet. The local Tibetan population is now outnumbered by Chinese immigrants who are given preferential treatment in education, jobs, and private enterprises.

If you want to know more or want to help support Tibetan charities, please visit the *website* of the Central Tibetan Administration (CTA), where the Tibetan people, under the leadership of His Holiness the Dalai Lama, have been carrying out a non-violent movement to regain their lost freedom and dignity.

IMPROVE YOUR SPIN TECHNIQUE TO REDUCE DIZZINESS AND NAUSEA

1. **Slow Down.** *Don't try and complete too many rotations too quickly. Allow your body time to get used to the motion.*

2. **Do Fewer Repetitions.** *Some people take six months or more to build up to the required 21 repetitions. Dizziness affects people differently regardless of their fitness level. I have taught yoga teachers & long-term yoga practitioners who experienced dizziness in the early stages of learning the Spin. Do only as many repetitions as you can without becoming uncomfortably dizzy. Gradually add repetitions over a period of weeks or even months until you can do the required 21 repetitions easily. Ensure all dizziness has disappeared (to prevent nausea) before moving onto Rite No. 2.*

3. **Continue To Build Repetitions Of Rites, 2, 3, 4, and 5** *in the recommended manner (3 repetitions in your first week, then add 2 per week until you are doing 21 repetitions in around ten weeks). Gradually increase the number of spins until you catch up with the other Rites.*

4. **Fine Tune Your Movement.** *Fine-tune your movement so it is smooth from head to toe. Steps that are too large, too small, too bouncy, or steps that start and stop instead of flowing from one to another create a motion of their own*

and contribute to dizziness. A smooth movement improves aerodynamics and reduces motion.

5. **Flat And Solid Level Surface.** *Do not spin on an uneven surface as this increases dizziness, and you will find it hard to keep your balance. Doing the Rites outside in nature is wonderful, but choose your surface carefully. Soft sand isn't suitable if you are going to try it on a beach.*

6. **Important – Keep Your Spin Movement Contained Within A Small, Obstacle Free Area.** *If you wander across the floor, slow down and adjust your movement. Bring your legs to hip-width apart and take small (not jerky) flowing steps. If you come into contact with an obstacle, avoid looking at it until you have stopped spinning and your dizziness has abated. Otherwise, you will feel very dizzy and may stagger or fall. In T5T, we carry out three special Energy Breaths after spinning. We place our hands on our hips and keep our eyes closed. You could try taking three deep, slow breaths instead.*

7. **Remember to Breathe!** *People often hold their breath while spinning, which reduces the oxygen supply to the brain and increases the likelihood of dizziness. Get into a habit of taking a breath before you begin spinning and constantly remind yourself to breathe normally while performing the Spin.*

ABOUT THE AUTHOR

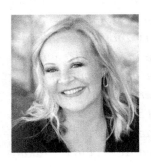

Carolinda Witt is an award-winning author who lives in Sydney.

She keeps herself fit and healthy by practicing The Five Tibetan Rites, which she began in 2000. Carolinda has taught the Rites to over 60,000 people worldwide through her books, online training course, DVD, and workshops – and attributes them to her youthful appearance and energetic outlook.

Carolinda highly recommends the Five Rites to anyone seeking a quick, easy, and effective daily exercise routine.

OTHER BOOKS, VIDEOS & ONLINE TRAINING COURSES BY THIS AUTHOR

Visit your favorite online retailer or the *T5T.com* website to discover other items by Carolinda Witt.

1) ONLINE TRAINING COURSE

- *Five Tibetan Rites Masterclass - Workbook & Video Series*

2) PAPERBACK & KINDLE BOOKS

1. *The Illustrated Five Tibetan Rites* – (UnMind Pty Ltd)
2. *The Eye of Revelation* – (UnMind Pty Ltd)

3) DVD

- *The Five Tibetans DVD Plus 2 x Bonus Training Manuals (PDF)* – UnMind Pty Ltd

4) LATEST BOOK

- *Double Agent Celery: MI5's Crooked Hero* – (Pen & Sword Books, UK)

Carolinda's grandfather married six times (two of them were mistresses.) He had six children to four different wives, most of whom knew nothing about the other and, in Carolinda's mother's case – about Dicketts himself. Sadly, Carolinda's mother died without ever knowing his name. Unable to tell her mother, Carolinda spent seven years researching and writing this book in her memory. What she discovered about Dicketts changed history and reunited a family.

Her grandfather, Walter Dicketts, an ex-RNAS officer, was recruited by MI5 and sent into Nazi Germany to infiltrate the German Secret Service in the guise of a traitor. If Dicketts succeeded, he was to extract crucial secrets about Germany's plans to invade Britain and communicate them back to MI5. With his life on the line, Dicketts managed to outwit his interrogators in Hamburg and Berlin before returning to Britain as, in the Nazi's eyes, a German spy. He didn't realize he had been betrayed before he even entered Germany.

- **Non-fiction prize** 2018 – Society of Women Writers
- *Wall Street Journal:* "Five Best Books About Clandestine Agents in WW11"

If you would like to let others know about the benefits of a regular Five Tibetans practice, please consider giving this book a review on *Amazon* or *Goodreads*. Thank you.

CONNECT WITH CAROLINDA WITT

I really appreciate you reading my book! Here are my social media coordinates:

1. *Connect with other Five Tibetans practitioners and me on my Facebook group – fivetibetanritesofrejuvenation*

2. *Visit my websites: www.t5t.com and carolindawitt.com*

3. *Visit my T5T blog and FAQ which has loads of interesting articles and information about practicing the Five Tibetan Rites and includes the latest research.*

Made in the USA
Columbia, SC
25 May 2024

35941816R00068